Immunity and Contagion: Transformations of Biopolitics in the Time of the Pandemic

Value Inquiry Book Series

VOLUME 416

Social Philosophy

The titles published in this series are listed at *brill.com/vibs* and *brill.com/socp*

Immunity and Contagion: Transformations of Biopolitics in the Time of the Pandemic

By

J. D. Mininger, Denis Petrina,
Aistis Žekevičius and Audronė Žukauskaitė

BRILL

LEIDEN | BOSTON

Cover illustration: Laisvydė Šalčiūtė, "(Melo)dramas. Kiss", 2015, oil, acrylic, canvas, 159x159 cm.

The Library of Congress Cataloging-in-Publication Data is available online at https://catalog.loc.gov

Typeface for the Latin, Greek, and Cyrillic scripts: "Brill". See and download: brill.com/brill-typeface.

ISSN 0929-8436
ISBN 978-90-04-74817-0 (hardback)
ISBN 978-90-04-74818-7 (e-book)
DOI 10.1163/9789004748187

This book is printed on acid-free paper and produced in a sustainable manner.

Contents

Acknowledgements

This monograph emanated as a result of a research project, "Immunity and Contagion: Transformations of Biopolitics in the Time of Pandemic," which took place between 2021 and 2024. The project has received funding from the Research Council of Lithuania (agreement no. S–MIP–21–36). The monograph also includes modified excerpts from previously published articles, which have been translated or rewritten. Audronė Žukauskaitė's article "Immunity and Symbiopolitics" appeared in the journal *Athena: filosofijos studijos*, no. 17, 2022, pp. 43–56. J. D. Mininger's article "Toward an Ethics of Dispossession: Philosophical Lessons from the Political Context of the COVID-19 Pandemic" was published in *Athena: filosofijos studijos*, no. 17, 2022, pp. 75–92. Denis Petrina's article "Sustojęs gyvenimas: pandemija ir afektyvieji sutrikimai" appeared in *Athena: filosofijos studijos*, no. 17, 2022, pp. 108–122. Aistis Žekevičius' article "Pandemic and Race: Un(fore)seen Circumstances, Same Old Biopolitics of Extraction and Use" was published in *Athena: filosofijos studijos*, no. 17, 2022, pp. 141–155. The authors would like to thank anonymous reviewers for their suggestions.

Introduction: Biopolitics in the Aftermath of the COVID-19 Pandemic

Audronė Žukauskaitė

This monograph explores the transformations of biopolitics in the aftermath of the COVID-19 pandemic. Not only pandemics but also simultaneously emerging war, migration, and climate crises make us rethink the very concept of biopolitics: the latter is no longer conceived of as an opposition between a sovereign power and a subjugated population but as an interaction between various social and political groups, ecological milieus, and habitats. Thus, in the face of these crises, the notion of biopolitics should be reconsidered and redefined not necessarily as a negative force but rather as a positive attempt to survey, govern, and overcome the crisis. We think that it is important to find new conceptual frameworks and philosophical concepts to define biopolitics in affirmative terms.

Among the first attempts to revisit the political and philosophical implications of the COVID-19 pandemic are Fernando Castrillón and Thomas Marchevsky's book *Coronavirus, Psychoanalysis, and Philosophy* (2021), Slavoj Žižek's *PANDEMIC!: COVID-19 Shakes the World* (2020) and *Pandemic 2: Chronicles of a Time Lost* (2021), Giorgio Agamben's *Where Are We Now? The Pandemic as Politics* (2021), Jean-Luc Nancy's *An All-Too-Human Virus* (2021), Benjamin Bratton's *The Revenge of the Real: Politics for a Post-pandemic World* (2021), as well as Judith Butler's book *What World Is This? A Pandemic Phenomenology* (2022) and Roberto Esposito's *Common Immunity: Biopolitics in the Age of the Pandemic* (2023). As stated by Žižek, the pandemic created contradictory expectations: on one hand, it resulted in even more rapid spreading of various ideological viruses, such as fake news, paranoid conspiracy theories, racism, and fundamentalism. However, Žižek hopes that another, more beneficent ideological virus will spread and, hopefully, infect us: "the virus of thinking of an alternate society, a society beyond nation-state, a society that actualizes itself in the forms of global solidarity and cooperation" (Žižek 2020: 39). Practices that emerged during the pandemic – those of volunteering, mutual help, and support (e.g., a universal basic income) – encourage us to think that the situation of crisis can potentially lead to novel forms of social organization and coexistence. As Jean-Luc Nancy points out, "In fact, the virus does communize us. It essentially puts us on a basis of equality, bringing us together in the need to make a common stand. […] Today we are reminded in every way of

 | DOI:10.1163/9789004748187_002

our togetherness, interdependence and solidarity" (Nancy 2022: 15–16). At the same time, the pandemic more acutely reveals and exacerbates the prevailing inequalities. As Judith Butler observes, these prevailing conditions include "environmental destruction, poverty, racism, global inequalities, and social violence, including violence directed against women and LGBTQI+ people" (Butler 2022: 1). The pandemic condition makes these inequalities more visible and intense, thus making us question the vision of a shared world. Perhaps, says Butler, we should think about different worlds, or even denounce the notion of the world for the sake of other, more inclusive notions, such as the planet.

But before discussing new philosophical concepts, let us examine what challenges the pandemic raises for the notion of biopolitics. From the very first days of the pandemic, philosophers were trying to apply the concept of biopolitics to the on-going events. On 26 February 2020, Agamben published his first text, "The Invention of an Epidemic," where he interpreted the government's attempts to manage the pandemic as a literal implementation of his theory of biopolitics. Agamben stated that the pandemic was invented (*sic!*) to introduce a state of exception and reduce populations to bare life. "The epidemic has made clear that the state of exception, to which our governments have actually accustomed us for quite some time, has become the normal condition. People are so used to living in conditions of perpetual crisis, that they seem not to realize that their lives have been reduced to a purely biological condition that has lost not only its political dimension, but also that of what is simply human" (Agamben 2021: 28). Agamben argues that the pandemic condition is used as a pretext to transform the paradigm of governance and suspend the constitutional guarantees to make the exception permanent. He even makes a comparison between the abolishment of the Weimar Constitution in Germany in 1933 and the recent security measures introduced by national governments. "We can use the term 'biosecurity' to describe the government apparatus that consists of this new religion of health, conjoined with the state power and its state of exception – an apparatus that is probably the most efficient of its kind that Western history has ever known" (Agamben 2021: 9). Such totalizing generalizations made by Agamben during the pandemic not only seem far-fetched but also risk compromising his theory of biopolitics.

The problem here is that Agamben blurs the distinction between the state of exception and the state of emergency. As Roberto Esposito observes, in some specific cases, like that of dictatorship, the state of emergency and the state of exception may converge but, in general, they refer to different intentions: the state of emergency aims to rebuild a normality interrupted by unforeseen events whereas the state of exception aims to break it for the sake of a different system (Esposito 2023: 169). Of course, it may be difficult to see the intentions behind these transformations. However, as Esposito explains, the essential question is whether the state is triggered by the power's "subjective will" or by an objective necessity. "Whatever one may say, a catastrophic flood or an earthquake is different from a political crisis or a foreign occupation. How can one deny that a pandemic is different from a *coup d'état,* even if it cannot be ruled out that the former might provoke the latter indirectly? [...] Without losing sight of possible analogies, the decision to restore the previous order through a series of emergency measures is different from that of using the unfavorable event to overthrow it" (Esposito 2023: 169–70). However, to claim, as Agamben did, that these limitations are exercised by a sovereign power to control and dominate populations is misleading and wrong. Of course, the limitations of individuals' rights may cause some risks to democracy; but perhaps the bigger risk comes from the opposite direction. As Esposito explains, the problem is not that a political power might shift toward sovereign dictatorship but that it is more likely to abandon its citizens, delegating all responsibilities to merely administrative regulations. "What we see emerging is not a return of the political, albeit in a sovereign version, but rather a depoliticization that brings to full fruition a tendency that has long been underway" (Esposito 2023: 172). The problem is not that biopolitical power controls too much but that it controls less and less by transposing all responsibilities to administrative government.

This decentralization of power, when the most pressing issues are handed to expert groups and administrators, puts the notion of biopolitics into question. As Nancy points out, all politics is biopolitics to the extent that it is always concerned with the life and health of populations and individuals. "It is for this reason that the term 'biopolitics,' which is used by many to stigmatize and disparage a politics assumed to interfere unduly with our lives, is an empty term. All societies have had to manage, at the very least, aspects of health, of birth rate, of food supply – but of course, this all depends on the state of knowledge and on that of ways of life. [...] There is no 'biopolitics' any more than there is a 'noopolitics' – but every politics has a way of managing health and knowledge ..." (Nancy 2022: 87–8). As Sergei Prozorov points out, the theories of biopolitics can teach us little about the pandemic because they seek to reveal something that is explicitly manifested. He makes an analogy with Freudian psychoanalysis which aims to interpret dreams, whatever their manifest content is, as the repressed form of sexual desires. But what about those dreams that are explicitly sexual? "By the same token, continues Prozorov, all politics (for Agamben) or modern politics (for Foucault and Esposito) is biopolitics, but what about the politics that is explicitly biopolitical in the sense of being preoccupied with the protection of human life against new viruses? [...] If theories of biopolitics teach us little about the pandemic and the pandemic teaches us little about biopolitics, what can we learn from this *obviously* biopolitical event that would not be so *obvious*?" (Prozorov 2022: 18–19). These questions force us to think if the notion of biopolitics is still relevant and what new theoretical twists it can take.

1 Biopolitics: A Historical Background

Although usually associated with Michel Foucault, the term "biopolitics" first appeared at the beginning of the twentieth century in the context of organistic and vitalistic theories of the state. As Esposito points out, the most influential references were Karl Binding's *Zum Werden und Leben der Staaten* (1920), Eberhard Dennert's *Der Staat als lebendiger Organismus* (1920), and Edward Hahn's *Der Staat, ein Lebenwesen* (1926). As Swedish political theorist Rudolph Kjellén points out, "This tension that is characteristic of life itself… pushed me to denominate such a discipline *biopolitics*, which is analogous with the science of life, namely, biology. […] Naming it in this way also expresses that dependence of the laws of life that society manifests and that promote, more than anything else, the state itself to that role of arbiter or at a minimum of mediator" (Kjellén 1920: 3–4, cited in the work of Esposito 2008: 17). In other words, instead of defining the state as the product of law and social contract, Kjellén sees the state as a living being, or a self-regulating organism.

Another source of biopolitical theory comes from comparative biology. The most important reference here is Jakob von Uexküll's *Staatsbiologie: Anatomie, Physiologie, Pathologie des Staates* (1920), where the state is defined in biological terms as a body with specific anatomy, physiology, and pathology. It is precisely the pathology of the state that is the main concern of his book: the body of the state is penetrated by "parasites," which should be cleansed by the state doctors. In this respect, the biopolitical rhetoric of Uexküll's book predicts the Nazi theory of degeneration, which would appear a decade later. Similar biopolitical ideas are expressed in Morley Roberts' *Bio-Politics: An Essay in the Physiology, Pathology and Politics of the Social and Somatic Organism*, published in 1938 in London. Roberts describes the state as an organism, comparing the defensive apparatus of the state with the immunity system of the body. Just as the bodily immune system rejects the foreign element, the state should reject the threatening elements of another race. We can see that Roberts' book predicts the racist biopolitics exploited during the period of National Socialism in Germany.

The racist biopolitics not only invented policies and regulations directed against actual racial threats but also supported the racist imagination concerning possible biological degeneration inflicted by so-called inferior races. The atrocities of genocide that resulted from this racist biopolitics were one of the reasons biopolitics disappeared for a while from the theoretical agenda. The theme of biopolitics reappears only in the 1960s in France but with quite a significant semantic reformulation. An example of this reformulation was Aroon Starobinski's *La biopolitique: Essai d'interprétation de l'histoire de l'humanité et des civilisations* (1960). As the title demonstrates, this book seeks to reformulate the question of biopolitics in the context of humanity and civilization, as if trying to neutralize the lethal consequences of biopolitical theory. As Esposito points out, "the concept of biopolitics thus risks being whittled down to the point of losing its meaning, that is, of being overturned into a sort of traditional humanism" (Esposito 2008: 20). Similar anthropological and humanistic indeterminacy was characteristic of Edgar Morin's *Introduction à une politique de l'homme* (1969), where biopolitics dissolves into the global ontology of the human being.

As we can see, the notion of biopolitics was initially explored in the contexts of political theory, geopolitics, comparative biology, and the history of ideas. With the texts of Michel Foucault, the concept acquired a philosophical meaning. The term appears in the first volume of the *History of Sexuality* (*The Will to Knowledge*), originally published in 1976, and in his lectures at the Collège de France in 1975–1979 (especially in the lecture of 17 March 1976, published in the volume *Society Must Be Defended*, 2003). Foucault was aware of the works of his predecessors, but he constructed his theory on completely new grounds. As Esposito points out, "Foucault's specific biopolitical perspective is indebted in the first place to Nietzschean genealogy" (Esposito 2008: 24). If political theories examine the relationship between individuals and power, which is external to them, Foucault interprets power as the multiplicity of forces which are immanent to the bodies of these individuals. It is the bodily or somatic dimension where power and the individual meet. In this respect, "life," or the biological dimension of the body, becomes the object of political manipulations. For Foucault, the notion of biopolitics is related to several political and social phenomena: first, biopolitics relates to a different articulation of sovereign power; second, it refers to governmentality as a new form of power; and third, it relates to racism as a strategy to exclude the surplus of economic overproduction (Lemke 2011: 34).

Foucault argues that starting from the seventeenth century, sovereign power evolved in two forms: first, power as a discipline directed towards an individual body (*anatomopolitics*), and second, *biopolitics* directed towards the population. On different scales, these technologies expressed "the two poles around which the organization of power over life was deployed" (Foucault 1998: 139).

With this rearrangement, the focus of power shifted from the power of death that characterized sovereign power to the power understood as regulation and management of life. As Foucault points out, the power of death was replaced by "the counterpart of a power that exerts a positive influence on life, that endeavors to administer, optimize, and multiply it, subjecting it to precise controls and comprehensive regulations" (Foucault 1998: 137). Foucault relates biopolitics as a "positive influence on life" to the emergence of capitalism and capitalist productive forces: "This bio-power was without question an indispensable element in the development of capitalism; the latter would not have been possible without the controlled insertion of bodies into the machinery of production and the adjustment of the phenomena of population to economic processes" (Foucault 1998: 140–41). Thus, power functions as a system of regulation and control, which arranges and connects political interests, economic incentives, and the living substance of the population into a multiple network of capitalist relationships. Foucault argues that political theory should be replaced by political economy to explain how life, productivity, and economic interests are related: "The adjustment of the accumulation of men to that of capital, the joining of the growth of human groups to the expansion of productive forces and the differential allocation of profit, were made possible in part by the exercise of bio-power in its many forms and modes of application. The investment of the body, its valorization, and the distributive management of its forces were at the time indispensable" (Foucault 1998: 141). In other words, the axiomatization of biological processes converted life into an economic category. Thus, the economic arrangement of life becomes compatible with liberal ideology and a new form of power called governmentality.

This second shape of biopolitics as governmentality involves the management of the population. Foucault argues that governmentality does not replace sovereign power and discipline but coexists with them to make the population disposable (Foucault 2007: 107–8). Foucault also reminds us that governmentality, which now has a political connotation, used to be related to problems of self-control, the wise government of house and family, and the pastoral government of souls. According to the ancient Greeks, the economy actually means the government of family life, and, therefore, this economic guidance perfectly expresses the essence of governmentality: "The essential issue of government will be the introduction of economy into political practice" (Foucault 2007: 95). This shift towards the economic model of government meant an important conceptual break: the government employs tactics rather than laws, and, therefore, the end and instruments of power are internal not to itself but to the things it governs (Foucault 2007: 99). Governmental power is immanent to the processes and bodies it intends to control. In this sense, Foucault's model of governmentality can be compared with Gilles Deleuze's notion of societies of control because control is a flexible and constantly changing system of measures that individuals are willing to accept as self-imposed order. This willingness is elucidated by the articulated nature of control: control functions not as a conspicuous form of power, but rather through immanent modulations, variations, and formations within the environment and networks. In essence, control achieves its effect through *naturalization*, rendering it imperceptible and sometimes even desirable to those under control. What distinguishes control from previous forms of (bio)power is its operational principle of *laissez-faire* – "not governing too much."

In this respect, the new art of government expresses the essence of liberal ideology: it is the manufacturing and consuming of freedom. However, the consumption of freedom cannot be unlimited, and thus, it has to invent limitations, measures of control, and security threats. As Foucault points out, "liberalism is an art of government that fundamentally deals with interests, and it cannot do this – and this is the other side of the coin – without at the same time managing the dangers and mechanisms of security/freedom…" (Foucault 2008: 66). Liberalism cannot proceed without the invention of a culture of danger and the need for security. The freedom to consume and the consumption of freedoms cannot be exploited without restriction because the resources are not limitless. Therefore, mechanisms for control should be invented to sort out which individuals are useful and productive and which can be excluded or abandoned.

Here, we come to the third aspect of biopolitics, that of racism. For Foucault, racism means not only the violence inflicted on some racial or ethnic group but also the inherently destructive function of the state that it directs against its elements that it deems useless or outright harmful. "It is primarily a way of introducing a break into the domain of life that is under power's control: the break between what must live and what must die" (Foucault 2003: 254). State racism establishes a caesura within a population itself, fragmenting and dividing the biological continuum. This means that the old sovereign's power to kill is delegated to the state now, and the state decides who is worthy or not worthy of living. In other words, racism transforms a political relationship into a biological relationship, exposing a non-useful and not-consumable element as a biological threat. As Foucault points out, "This is not, then, a military, warlike, or political relationship, but a biological relationship. And the reason this mechanism can come into play is that the enemies who have to be done away with are not adversaries in the political sense of the term; they are threats, either external or internal, to the population and for the population" (Foucault 2003: 255–6). The invention of danger or threat expresses the essence of a control society and legitimates the repressive function of the state.

Interestingly, this securitarian apparatus not only manifests in the present reality but also, and more importantly, in the realm of potentiality. In this context, Brian Massumi's concept of "ontopower," defined as a preemptive mode of power that "converts a future, virtual cause into a taking-actual-effect in the present" (Massumi 2015: 16), is particularly relevant. Massumi argues that ontopower "must move as the accident moves, to where it may erupt, catching it before it actually emerges" (Massumi 2015: 40), emphasizing how it operates by anticipating and intercepting potential threats before they materialize. This dynamic was especially evident during the pandemic, where preventive and prognostic measures were employed not only to mitigate but essentially to preempt the detrimental effects of the virus. Such a *modus operandi* underscores the need to expand the notion of securitarian biopolitics beyond mere bureaucratic governmentality and population management to encompass the creation and control of living conditions and emergent situations. Massumi aptly observes that "ontopower exceeds and encompasses other modes, even biopower" (Massumi 2015: 234–235). This observation encapsulates a formidable challenge for theorizing the pandemic within the present frameworks of biopolitics.

2 Negative or Affirmative Biopolitics?

Foucault's notion of biopolitics covers many insights and aspects which continue to influence contemporary thought. In recent research on biopolitics, we can discern three main tendencies in interpreting Foucault's ideas: political theology, political economy, and posthumanism (Žukauskaitė, Wilmer 2016). The first tendency, which evolves from Foucault's writing on racism and the function of the state, is represented by Giorgio Agamben. Relating Foucault's critique of state racism to recent phenomena, such as the War on Terror, Agamben argues that a biopolitical caesura is at work not only in totalitarian states but also in so-called liberal democracies. Biological caesura is legitimated by the state of exception, which, according to Carl Schmitt, is the main function of sovereignty. Following Schmitt, Agamben defines the sovereign as someone who decides on the state of exception: it is a moment when normal jurisdiction is suspended, and the living beings, who used to be protected by the law, now become abandoned (Agamben 2005: 1). Agamben claims that the state of exception, which usually refers to such exceptional situations as civil war, insurrection, or resistance, becomes a permanent paradigm of government in contemporary politics. From this perspective, claims Agamben, there is no essential difference between totalitarian and democratic states: "In this sense, modern totalitarianism can be defined as the establishment, by means of the state of exception, of a legal civil war that allows for the physical elimination not only of political adversaries but of entire categories of citizens who for some reason cannot be integrated into the political system. Since then, the voluntary creation of a permanent state of emergency [...] has become one of the essential practices of contemporary states, including so-called democratic ones" (Agamben 2005: 2). The paradigmatic example of the state of exception is the concentration camp, where the law is suspended, and bare lives are produced. Agamben argues that the structure of the camp is "the hidden matrix of the politics in which we are still living" (Agamben 1998: 175) and that the same structure reproduces itself in detention camps, migration centers, and other zones of juridical indistinction. As was mentioned before, Agamben believes that some measures applied by local governments during the pandemic, such as social distancing or quarantine, present another form of the state of exception, which expresses the new religion of health conjoined with the state power.

Not only Agamben's reaction to the pandemic but his entire project of biopolitics received a substantial critique. First, Agamben is criticised for relying on the juridical model of power – Agamben thinks that it is the law and its reformulations (like the state of exception) that introduce the biological caesura between *bios* and *zoē*, between legally approved life and bare life. He traces contemporary reconfigurations of law to the sources of antiquity, however, often ignoring the historical differences between contemporary jurisdiction and the understanding of law in antiquity. As Lemke observes, "Agamben's attempt to correct and amend Foucault [...] also abandons the latter's central insight, namely, that biopolitics is a historical phenomenon that cannot be separated from the development of modern states, the emergence of the human sciences, and the formation of capitalist relations of production. Without the biopolitical project's necessary placement within a historical-social context, 'bare life' becomes an abstraction whose complex conditions of emergence must remain as obscure as its political implications" (Lemke 2011: 63). Agamben not only ignores the historical differences between the notions of law in antiquity, modernity, and contemporaneity but also departs from Foucault's analysis of power. Foucault was interested in the "microphysics of power" and the ways it penetrates and creates social norms and individuals. Foucault thinks that power is always immanent in the social production of normality, whereas Agamben depicts power as an obscure and negative transcendence, following the tradition of negative theology. As Lemke points out, "Agamben's analysis remains in thrall to the law and owes more to Carl Schmitt than it does to Foucault. If Schmitt situates sovereign power in its ability to call for a state of exception and a suspension of rights [...], Foucault is interested in normal conditions, which exist below, next to, and partially counter to legal mechanisms. Whereas Schmitt is interested in how the norm is suspended, Foucault is concerned with the production of normality" (Lemke 2011: 60). After all, biopolitics is concerned with the management of life rather than the production of death.

Another problem with Agamben's approach is that he concentrates exclusively on the role of the state as if the state has a particular concern to suppress and eliminate individuals. Such an understanding of biopolitics is exclusively negative and difficult to explain in the context of the capitalist mode of production. As was said before, it was Foucault who stated that the emergence of biopolitics comes together with the formation and development of the capitalist mode of production. In Lemke's opinion, the biggest shortcoming of Agamben's theory is that he does not realize that biopolitics is essentially a political economy of life (Lemke 2011: 60). Thus, Agamben's interpretations derive biopolitics from a negative quasi-transcendent power and in this sense preclude any actual alternative. As Antonio Negri states, "These interpretations offer an understanding of biopolitics that creates an uncertain, dangerous, even destructive magma, a tendency that turns much more towards thanatopolitics than a true political affirmation of life" (Negri 2008: 15). Michael Hardt and Antonio Negri also criticize Agamben for not looking for positive alternatives that can be linked to new forms of political subjectivity and resistance.

To this negative concept of biopolitics, Hardt and Negri juxtapose an affirmative, positive interpretation of biopolitics, which derives the new political subjectivity and the power of resistance from the individuals' capacity for labor. In other words, the production of subjectivity is understood here as the subjectivity that produces. Hardt and Negri, along with Paolo Virno and Maurizio Lazzarato, thus represent the second trend, that of political economy, in which resistance to power is linked to labor power and new forms of collaboration and production. As Virno points out, "to comprehend the rational core of the term 'bio-politics', we should begin with a different concept, a much more complicated concept from a philosophical standpoint: that of *labor-power*. [...] What does 'labor-power' mean? It means *potential* to produce" (Virno 2004: 81). It is no coincidence that biopolitics emerges precisely at this moment when the capitalist mode of production takes place – the "vital" interest of biopolitics is not annihilation and death but living labor. "The living body becomes an object to be governed not for its intrinsic value, but because it is the substratum of what really matters: labor-power as the aggregate of the most diverse human faculties… For this reason, and this reason alone, it is legitimate to talk about 'bio-politics'" (Virno 2004: 83). To distance themselves from the negative concept of biopolitics, Hardt and Negri propose a distinction between biopower and biopolitical production: "Biopower stands above society, transcendent, as a sovereign authority and imposes its order. Biopolitical production, in contrast, is immanent to society and creates social relationships and forms through collaborative forms of labor" (Hardt, Negri 2004: 94–5). Hardt and Negri believe that biopolitical production in its broadest sense – which includes not only labor relations but also the creation of communication networks, affects, discourses, and forms of life – creates a power of a different kind that can resist the pressures of biopower. "The perspective of resistance makes clear the difference between these two powers: the biopower against which we struggle is not comparable in its nature or form to the power of life by which we defend and seek our freedom" (Hardt, Negri 2009: 57). If biopower is defined as a power that seeks to control life, then biopolitics defines the power of life to resist and create new forms of subjectivity.

Hardt and Negri trace the antinomy of biopower and biopolitics to Spinoza's distinction between *potestas* and *potentia*: *potestas* is a coercive, external power that presses us from above, whereas *potentia* is the potentiality of the being itself, which can manifest itself through labor or any other creative activity. The operation of biopower or *potestas* is embodied by the empire, which we can interpret as a new form of government, whereas biopolitical potentiality is revealed by the multitude – a new political subject – which resists the pressure of power (Hardt, Negri 2000; 2004). In other words, there is an eternal antinomy between *potestas* and *potentia*, biopower and biopolitical production, capital and labor. In this sense, biopolitical production and biopower can never be cleanly separated. Taking this into account, Negri argues that "the antinomy of the two effects (that is, the two characters) of potency cannot be defined as ontological dualism: it is a contrast that never ceases self-producing, a conflict that continuously takes place and is continuously resolved and immediately re-forms at another level" (Negri 2013: 25). In this sense, biopolitical production and biopower can be seen as two tendencies or directions in the production of subjectivities.

The contradictory nature of biopolitics is also revealed in Roberto Esposito's works. Esposito examines biopolitics both as a negative sovereign power and as a form of communal life: the essence of biopolitics lies in the individuals' choice between the need to protect their immunity against political others and the attempt to be a part of a political community. Both immunity (*immunitas*) and community (*communitas*) derive from the Latin word *munus*, which refers to "office" – a task, obligation, or duty (Esposito 2011: 5). Thus, immunity would imply someone who performs no office and who is exempted from the obligation of the *munus*, whereas community is based precisely on this obligation. In this respect, community is always struggling to keep its boundaries and protect itself from "others"; on the contrary, without these "others," community would lose its meaning. Esposito is trying to solve this aporia by relating the social, political, and juridical notion of immunity to biological immunity: in biology, the immune system acts both as a defensive or reactionary boundary and as a positive collaborative network. Esposito states that the notion of collective immunity (or "herd immunity"), which was praised and emphasized so much during the pandemic, will allow us to connect biopolitics with a broader social and political context and conceptualize new forms of communal subjectivity.

Another attempt to rethink the theory of biopolitics is related to the emergence of new directions in philosophy. These directions include posthumanism, indigenous cosmologies, new materialism, speculative realism, animal and plant studies, and others. What all these philosophical frameworks have in common is a disbelief in universal humanity and a universal human knowledge, based on dark and often concealed mechanisms of appropriation, colonization, and objectification of human and nonhuman others and natural environments. This change in perspective requires a new notion of biopolitics, which takes into account not only liberal individuals but also more-than-human others. This new approach should embrace *zoē* as a positive life force which is distributed in humans, animals, plants, matter and different habitats. As Rosi Braidotti insists, this new direction "goes beyond Foucault's idea of the biopolitical in that it implies a notion of subjectivity as vital and self-organizing matter, an embedded form of 'matter-realism' that is intrinsically connected to the posthuman definition of Life as *zoē,* or a dynamic and generative nonhuman force" (Braidotti 2016: 33). The main discrepancy between Foucault's notion of biopolitics and the posthumanist approach has to do with the displacement of humanism and anthropocentrism. Such an approach withdraws from the humanist model of "Man" based on "the Eurocentric, masculinist universalism that is still operative in most knowledge production scientific systems" (Bignall, Braidotti 2019: 2). By contrast, posthumanism offers perspectival "situated knowledge," which takes into account feminism, gender theory, postcolonialism, and emerging indigenous philosophies. This new approach also opposes anthropocentrism and human exceptionalism, based on species hierarchy and exclusion of nonhuman others. It explores the entanglements between human and nonhuman others and discusses their shared vulnerability and precarity. As Braidotti points out, "Life is not the prerogative of humans only, it opens up a *zoē*-political or post-anthropocentric dimension. This inaugurates both a negative or reactive form of panhuman planetary bond, which recomposes humanity around a commonly shared bond of vulnerability, and also new modes of connection between humans and the other species" (Braidotti 2016: 46). In this context, the question of biopolitics and biopower is still pertinent; however, the scope of its applicability has moved beyond the premises articulated by Foucault.

3 Planetary Biopolitics?

The experience of the pandemic gave even stronger impulse to rethink our relationships with more-than-human others and the environment: humans' intrusion into natural ecosystems, as well as the destruction and commercialization of other species, is directly related to ever-present epidemics and the emergence of so-called zoonotic viruses. Benjamin Bratton maintains that the concept of biopolitics must encompass not only other people (even though it is critically important to speak about structural inequality, poverty, and geographical differences) but also other species, the environment, and the atmosphere. In other words, he insists on a need to create "a *positive biopolitics at planetary scale*" (Bratton 2021: 30). Therefore, biopolitics must be centered not around biopower that disciplines individuals and manages populations but around the notion of governmentality that monitors and surveys ecosystems. Even though the term "surveillance" has negative connotations and covers almost all flaws of capitalist technocratic societies, Bratton interprets the term as a technology that is necessary for sensing, modeling, and predicting social phenomena.

Planetary biopolitics implies not only the direct governance of the ecosystem but also requires reconsidering relationships between the individual and society. It is important to point out that Foucault's notion of biopolitics was based on the ideas of liberal individualism: "Foucault's account of the history of subjectivity, identity, and individuation is also a history of liberal individualism, a set of presumptions deep within diverse philosophical and popular political commitments" (Bratton 2021: 67). In other words, it is based on the assumption that first and foremost, we are individuals who may or may not enter into relationships with other individuals. In this respect, surveillance and control are seen as the infringement of individual autonomy. However, post-pandemic politics reveals not only our dependency on others but also the necessity to engage in collective modes of social existence. As Bratton observes, "Each organism is a transmission medium for information – from ideas to viruses – and is defined by who and what each is connected to and disconnected from. The political premise of 'immunization' – to make oneself immune by excluding someone or someone else – must be couched in conceptual and technical models of the social that are as inclusive and agnostic as epidemiological models and which carry the same weight of shared responsibility" (Bratton 2021: 34). The immunological principle of vaccination demonstrates that individual immunity contributes to collective immunity and vice versa: collective immunity minimizes the risk for an individual. This is the positive task of post-pandemic biopolitics: "Those politics will need to remap and deconflate identity, subjectivity, status, and agency from one another in order to build the co-immunological commons" (Bratton 2021: 65). Esposito comes to the same conclusion by pointing out that "What appeared to be a paradigmatic opposition – between *communitas* and *immunitas* – was suddenly revealed during the pandemic to be what it has always been, that is, a dialectic in which one term is indistinguishable from the other" (Esposito 2023: 185). Unfortunately, these new modes of positive biopolitics do not preclude the negative ones, which reappear again and create new lines of separation and exclusion.

Planetary biopolitics also requires us to rethink the premises of human domination and the effects of globalization and acceleration. The pandemic experience explicitly reveals the interdependence between humans, animals, and viruses. As Dipesh Chakrabarty observes, "The current moment of the COVID-19 pandemic belongs not only to the global history of capitalism and its destructive impact on human life, but it also represents a moment in the history of biological life on this planet when humans are acting as the *amplifiers* of a virus…" (Chakrabarty 2020). The great acceleration and human mobility created new opportunities not only for humans but also for viruses – they can jump species and use humans as agents for their mobility. This means that pandemics and epidemics are the result of increasing human activity, and they have accompanied humans ever since the beginning of agriculture and the domestication of animals. Chakrabarty refers to David M. Morens et al.'s observation that "Human beings are the ultimate causes of the pandemics. […] Deforestation, agricultural intensification, urbanization, and ecosystem disruption bring people into contact with wildlife and their potentially zoonotic pathogens" (Morens et al. 2020). All these anthropogenic interventions, known as the Anthropocene, have lethal consequences for the human population that still has to compete for its survival in the Darwinian history of life and offer new opportunities for viruses, which have more and more chances to adapt and multiply.

This new virological condition, as Chakrabarty observes, should change our notion of biopolitics, which remains oriented towards sovereign power and does not take into account the effects of globalization. "This gives us a glimpse into the ironical nature of the crisis of the biopolitical that we are living through. Bio-power, as Foucault formulated it, was about securitizing human life. Health, food, and housing are part of it. But the frenzied expansion of bio-power over the last several decades – the great acceleration of human history – has undone that security. [...] Yet we debate only bio-power and sovereignty – as if the virus could still be contained within the phatic ..." (Chakrabarty 2023: 37–38). The problem here is that we continue debating biopolitics in terms of sovereignty and bio-power without noticing that the terms are not relevant anymore. Human life and politics should be studied not as a unique and autonomous phenomenon but as a chapter in the geobiology and the deep history of the planet. "Bio" makes only one component in the complexity of life, therefore, biopolitics should be "provincialized" or put in a "minoritarian" mode. "We would wonder if it were possible for humanity as a whole to look on themselves as a 'minor' form of life and work toward minoritarian forms of political thought, of the kind that Arendt or Deleuze on Kafka have educated us in, thoughts that would want to avoid 'majoritarian' [...] dreams of domination" (Chakrabarty 2023: 39). Similarly, Bruno Latour (2021a; 2021b) argues that we should stop speaking about humans and human politics and refer instead to terrestrials (the earthbound) that would not prioritize humans and take into account other species. "Saying 'We are earthbound, we are terrestrials amid terrestrials' *does not lead to the same politics as saying* 'We are humans in nature'. The two are not made of the same cloth – or rather of the same mud" (Latour 2018: 86). This implies a new notion of (bio)politics that would require the emergence of a new ecological class (Latour, Schultz 2022) that would take into account the conditions of habitability.

Bearing all these philosophical interventions in mind, it becomes apparent that the concept of biopolitics must be radically revisited and linked not only with the possibilities of an alternative political order but also with planetary conditions of habitability. Biopolitics should be understood not as a negative force (although it still retains its power to make differences and exclusions) but as a positive affirmative potentiality. Such kind of biopolitics should take into account all human populations and groups, including the underprivileged, the dispossessed, the precarious, migrants and refugees, and indigenous first nations. It should take responsibility for all injustice done to human and nonhuman others, to our environment and habitats, including climate change. This gesture requires a new conceptuality that allows us to comprehend the new alliances between organic and inorganic components. Instead of discussing the opposition between a sovereign power and an oppressed individual, we should examine mixed states: assemblages, consortiums, symbionts, holobionts, hybrids, and chimeras. Instead of discussing *develop-*

ment as a constant production and growth, we should converse about *envelopment* (Latour, Schultz 2022) and entanglement with our habitats. All these reconsiderations urge us to rethink critically the notion of biopolitics and propose new modes of biopolitics that will resonate with our posthuman and post-pandemic planetary condition.

4 The Outline of Chapters

The monograph consists of two distinct yet interconnected parts. "Biopolitics and Pandemic: Vulnerability, Deprivation, Dispossession" aims to examine the negative effects of the pandemic. It is obvious that the pandemic has triggered many ideological viruses which were implicitly characteristic to our societies: fake news, conspiracy theories, explosions of racism, inequality and violence. Thus, the first part of the monograph examines these negative effects of dispossession, affective disorders, and racial violence. However, the experience of the pandemic also encourages us to think about alternative forms of society. Therefore, the second part of the book "Post-pandemic Biopolitics: Subjectivities, Spatialities, Temporalities" outlines a new kind of biopolitics, namely, planetary biopolitics. It reconceptualizes new modes of subjectivity, such as "collective immunity," or "the transindivdual." It also highlights the need for new posthuman epistemology and a new methodological approach that would allow us to observe and monitor human and nonhuman interactions on a planetary scale.

The monograph starts with J. D. Mininger's article "Philosophy as Immunity and Contagion," which challenges the idea that the COVID-19 pandemic made people more philosophical, as proposed by Jean Grondin. While the pandemic may have prompted deeper reflection and self-inquiry in some individuals, the chapter expresses severe doubts over the effectiveness of philosophical inquiry as an immunization against false discourse and prejudice, as seeking truth through philosophical inquiry may not necessarily lead to genuine self-awareness or a risk-taking process of self-inquiry that challenges existing beliefs and assumptions. Deploying Karl Jaspers' concept of a "limit situation" to consider these matters and analyzing Plato's famous account of the death of Socrates as a foundational historical and conceptual moment for philosophy, the author further problematizes the metaphor of philosophy as an inoculation against false discourse by suggesting that philosophy should be first and foremost concerned not about finding solace in the face of suffering but about engaging in rigorous truth-seeking even in the most challenging circumstances. By reminding the reader(s) that the task of philosophy lies in the pursuit of truth rather than the possession of it, J. D. Mininger seemingly comes to terms with the idea that truth always remains just out of reach, whereas philosophy itself embodies an "essential position of otherness," as Foucault would have it, and requires a willingness to embrace uncertainty and ambiguity in the time marked by limit(ing) and liminal shifts.

Denis Petrina's article "Total Lockdown: the Pandemic and Affective Disorders" delves into the intricate relationship between the pandemic governmentality and individual and collective affects in times of crisis. It contends that while the initial focus on public health and population security was crucial, it often disregarded psychosomatic well-being and existential uncertainties and insecurities, essentially blurring the line between care and control. The pursuit of security, both politically and discursively (referred to as the "sanitizing discourse"), inevitably homogenized a wide spectrum of affective responses, predominantly negative, within normative discursive frameworks. The chapter argues that this approach is reductionist and advocates for a deeper and more nuanced understanding of lived experiences beyond statistical data and medical terminology. By drawing parallels between affect and virus as contagions, it aims to transcend the confines of the "discursive lockdown" and, amidst "sad passions," emphasizes shared vulnerability as a catalyst for affirmative affects like resilience, hope, and care. Through an exploration of individual and collective (para)discursive practices – from emerging grassroots communities to creative coping mechanisms – the chapter endeavors to reimagine social dynamics and collective affects amidst the challenges posed by the pandemic. Ultimately, it raises a crucial question about resisting the constraints imposed by the "sanitizing discourse" through communal care.

In examining the nexus of race and the COVID-19 pandemic, Aistis Žekevičius' "Pandemic and Race: Un(fore)seen Circumstances, Same Old Biopolitics?" renders a complex interplay between the two, revealing deep-seated structural inequalities and necropolitical dynamics in play. By suggesting to treat the logic of race as a lens through which bodies are categorized, populations are rendered disposable, and existing hierarchies are reinforced, the chapter focuses on the all-encompassing capitalization of life that neoliberal biopolitics entails, therefore privileging economic considerations over human value and exacerbating differential vulnerability. As Aistis Žekevičius shows, the predicament is further aggravated by the colonial epistemic undertones of epidemiology, which continue to haunt us by perpetuating global health disparities and reinforcing racialized categorizations of difference, whereas the situational nature of vulnerability magnifies risks for marginalized communities in times of crisis, further exposing systemic injustices. And while remedies proposed by the author include decolonial awareness, socio-economic restructuring, ecological restoration, and solidarity, their implementation remains elusive. Despite shifts in global focus from the pandemic to other pressing issues, systemic racism persists, indicating the necessity of a paradigmatic shift towards recognizing universal human interconnectedness and affirming the value of each individual's life, irrespective of race. In a way, this allows us to reconsider how the pandemic unveils enduring challenges and calls for transformative action to dismantle entrenched inequities and foster a more inclusive and just society.

Another contribution by J. D. Mininger, "Toward an Ethics of Dispossession: Philosophical Lessons from the Political Context of the COVID-19 Pandemic," offers an exploration of the intersection of mourning, critical reflexivity, and Foucauldian critique in the context of pandemic politics, emphasizing the importance of challenging power structures, advocating for ethical responses to the crisis. Imbued with critical reflexivity, the intricate process of mourning prompts an interrogation of power dynamics determining who is deemed worthy of it and who is not. Judith Butler's insights underscore the necessity of mourning as a means of identifying with suffering while critically evaluating the normative violence inherent in societal structures, whereas Michel Foucault's concept of critique, rooted in Kantian enlightenment ideals, advocates for ongoing self-transformation and resistance to dominant power structures. The author suggests that this critical ethos, aligned with virtue, challenges uncritical obedience, and demands a reevaluation of governmentality and subjectivity in pandemic politics. By employing critical reflexivity and Foucauldian notion of critique in his reconsideration of mourning, J. D. Mininger formulates a call to action to subvert dominant narratives, resist normative violence, and foster a more equitable and just response to the pandemic's complexities.

The second part of the monograph, "Post-pandemic Biopolitics: Subjectivities, Spatialities, Temporalities," is mainly concerned with the formulation of new principles of biopolitics that would help us navigate the complexities highlighted by the pandemic challenges. These include but are by no means limited to the shift towards posthuman epistemology that anticipates the emergence of a posthuman genealogy, the move towards transindividual understanding of biopolitics where differences and heterogeneities result in affirmative alliances. It also suggests the need to reconsider the human dominance over the Earth's ecosystems that asks for a new planetary biopolitical paradigm that embraces interconnectedness and sustainability. This leads to an affirmative model of biopolitics that challenges the traditional opposition between immunity and community.

Denis Petrina's article "The Death of Man: The Post-pandemic Condition?" advocates for a reassessment of humanity's epistemological status using Foucault's insights as a guide. By examining the pandemic's philosophical implications through the lenses of the body, biopolitics, and the subject, the paper reconsiders the body's limits and its entanglement with others (e.g., viruses), highlighting the pandemic's revelation of intrinsic bodily fragility, vulnerability, and interconnectivity. This prompts a reevaluation of the boundaries of human autonomy and agency, exemplified by the COVID-19 pandemic's challenge to traditional political ontologies and the subsequent need for a posthuman epistemology to navigate its complexities within the context of biopolitical management. Consequently, the pandemic shifts the discourse from human-centered biopolitics to a broader consideration of life itself. The chapter concludes by proposing a genealogy of the post-pandemic subject, grounded in a posthuman reinterpretation of Foucault's concept of "technologies of the self" that acknowledges human vulnerability and interdependence with multiple others. It envisions the emergence of a posthuman genealogy that transcends conventional notions of the human subject, reflecting the ongoing evolution of post-pandemic biopolitical discourse.

In "Transindividual Biopolitics," Audronė Žukauskaitė suggests rethinking the notion of biopolitics by introducing the concept of the transindividual. The term "transindividual" was suggested by Gilbert Simondon to refer to one of the stages of the process of human individuation. For him, the subject is a system of three successive stages of being: the pre-individual phase, the individuated phase, and the transindividual phase. Following Simondon, Balibar argues that the pandemic creates new forms of transindividuality when a human individual is related to pre-individual potential, namely, a virus, and, at the same time, to a transindividual condition, such as "common immunity." This allows us to introduce a new type of transindividual biopolitics that unifies everyone as a specimen of the human species. In other words, besides "conventional biopolitics," which is still potent and incessantly introduces differences between different sub-species, we can discern a transindividual biopolitics whose field of operation is not the individual but the transindividual community, forming alliances with nonhuman viruses and transhuman technologies.

Aistis Žekevičius' chapter "Post-pandemic Biopolitics: Reconciling the Geological, the Global, and the Planetary" raises a number of questions regarding the viability of biopolitics in post-pandemic times, setting the stage for a nuanced exploration of diverse theoretical frameworks that encompasses both the spatial and the temporal. At its core, however, the inquiry poses fundamental questions regarding the universality of liveability and resource distribution in a post-pandemic world by highlighting the entanglement of geological forces with racialization processes. Building on Kathryn Yusoff's geological critique and Elizabeth A. Povinelli's notion of geontopower, Žekevičius takes their critique of the popular conception of the Anthropocene as the springboard to challenge traditional distinctions between life and nonlife, and advocate for a reevaluation of human dominance over the Earth's ecosystems. Furthermore, the author's engagement with Dipesh Chakrabarty's notion of planetary anthropologies allows him to interrogate the boundaries between human and nonhuman scales of thinking, and further stresses the need for a reexamination of humanity's relationship with the biosphere. In synthesizing these diverse perspectives, the chapter underscores the urgency of forging a new biopolitical paradigm capable of transcending anthropocentric worldviews and embracing the interconnectedness of all forms of life on the Earth. The pursuit of equitable and sustainable planetary biopolitics, though, still demands a coordinated effort to bridge theory and practice, which would enable us to chart a course toward a more harmonious coexistence within our shared planetary ecosystem.

In "Immunity and Symbiopolitics," Audronė Žukauskaitė discusses the relationships between biopolitics and the notion of immunity. The notion of immunity is the perfect metaphor for biopolitical government. Similar to the immune system, which fights everything that it sees as "nonself," biopolitical power discriminates against what it sees as "different" or "other." However, recent research in immunology reveals that, besides its defensive reaction towards an external, contagious element, the immune system also has a positive function. As Alfred I. Tauber suggested, immunity should be seen as an ecological system that not simply reacts toward the external element but negotiates between the "self" and "nonself" within the system. This model of ecological immunology is also a good methodological tool to rethink the notion of biopolitics: instead of seeing biopolitics as the opposition between a sovereign power and an oppressed individual, we can interpret it as a network of sympoietic interactions between individuals, technologies, and nonhuman others. Such an affirmative model of symbiopolitics reframes the opposition between immunity and community. To acquire immunity, I do not have to protect the "self" from "nonself" or "other"; on the contrary, the "other" is what makes "my" immunity possible. In this model, differences and heterogeneities are not rejected or suppressed but are transformed affirmatively, so that they produce sympoietic alliances. The final chapter, "Conclusions: Toward a Planetary Biopolitics," summarizes all chapters and outlines the contours of planetary biopolitics.

References

Agamben, Giorgio. 1998. *Homo Sacer: Sovereign Power and Bare Life*, translated by Daniel Heller-Roazen. Stanford, CA: Stanford University Press.

Agamben, Giorgio. 2005. *State of Exception*, translated by Kevin Attell. Chicago: University of Chicago Press.

Agamben, Giorgio. 2021. *Where Are We Now? The Epidemic as Politics*, translated by Valeria Dani, London: Eris.

Bignall, Simone and Rosi Braidotti, Rosi. 2019. "Posthuman Systems", in *Posthuman Ecologies: Complexity and Process After Deleuze*, eds. Rosi Braidotti and Simone Bignall, New York, London: Rowman and Littlefield, pp. 1–16.

Binding, Karl. 1920. *Zum Werden und Leben der Staaten: Zehn Staatsrechtliche Abhandlungen*. Munich and Leipzig: Duncker & Humblot.

Braidotti, Rosi. 2016. "Posthuman Affirmative Politics", in *Resisting Biopolitics: Philosophical, Political and Performative Strategies*, eds. S. E. Wilmer and Audronė Žukauskaitė, New York, London: Routledge, pp. 30–56.

Bratton Benjamin. 2021. *The Revenge of the Real: Politics for a Post-pandemic World*. London, New York: Verso.

Butler, Judith. 2002. "What Is Critique? an Essay on Foucault's Virtue", in Ingram, D. (ed.). *The Political: Readings in Continental Philosophy*. London: Basil Blackwell.

Butler, Judith. 2004. *Precarious Life*. New York: Verso.

Butler, Judith. 2020. "Judith Butler: Mourning is a Political Act Amid the Pandemic and Its Disparities. Interview with George Yancy". Published in Truthout. April 30, 2020, https://truthout.org/articles/judith-butler-mourning-is-a-political-act-amid-the-pandemic-and-its-disparities/. Accessed 2 February 2024.

Butler Judith. 2022. *What World Is This? A Pandemic Phenomenology*, New York: Columbia University Press.

Castrillón, Fernando and Marchevsky, Thomas (eds.). 2021. *Coronavirus, Psychoanalysis, and Philosophy: Conversations on Pandemics, Politics, and Society*, London and New York: Routledge.

Chakrabarty, Dipesh. 2018. *The Crises of Civilization: Exploring Global and Planetary Histories*. Oxford: Oxford University Press.

Chakrabarty, Dipesh. 2020. "An Era of Pandemics? What Is Global and What Is Planetary About COVID-19", *Critical Inquiry*, October 2020, https://critinq.wordpress.com/2020/10/16/an-era-of-pandemics-what-is-global-and-what-is-planetary-about-covid-19/. Accessed 22 February 2024.

Chakrabarty, Dipesh. 2021. *The Climate of History in a Planetary Age*. Chicago: The University of Chicago Press.

Chakrabarty, Dipesh. 2023. "Foreword". In: *New Earth Histories: Geo-Cosmologies and the Making of the Modern World*. Chicago, London: University of Chicago Press.

Chakrabarty, Dipesh. 2023. *One Planet, Many Worlds. The Climate Parallax*. Waltham, Mass.: Brandeis University Press.

Dennert, Eberhard. 1920. *Der Staat als lebendiger Organismus: Biologische Betrachtungen zum Aufbau der neuen Zeit*. Halle: C. E. Müller.

Esposito, Roberto. 2008. *Bíos: Biopolitics and Philosophy*, translated by Timothy Campbell. Minneapolis: University of Minnesota Press.

Esposito, Roberto. 2011. *Immunitas: The Protection and Negation of Life*, translated by Zakiya Hanafi, Cambridge: Polity Press.

Esposito, Roberto. 2023. *Common Immunity: Biopolitics in the Age of the Pandemic*, translated by Zakiya Hanafi, Cambridge: Polity Press.

Foucault, Michel. 1993. "About the Beginning of the Hermeneutics of the Self: Two Lectures at Dartmouth", *Political Theory* 21 (2): 198–227.

Foucault, Michel. 1998. *The History of Sexuality, Vol 1: The Will to Knowledge*, translated by Robert Hurley. London: Penguin.

Foucault, Michel. 2003. *Society Must Be Defended: Lectures at the Collège de France, 1975–1976*, translated by David Macey. London: Penguin.

Foucault, Michel. 2007. *Security, Territory, Population: Lectures at the Collège de France, 1977–1978*, translated by Graham Burchell. New York: Palgrave Macmillan.

Foucault, Michel. 2007. "What Is Critique?", in *The Politics of Truth*. New York: Semiotexte.

Foucault, Michel. 2008. *The Birth of Biopolitics: Lectures at the Collège de France, 1978–79*, translated by Graham Burchell. New York: Palgrave Macmillan.

Foucault, Michel. 2010. *The Government of Self and Others: Lectures at the Collège de France 1982–1983*. London: Palgrave MacMillan.

Grondin, Jean. 2022. "How a Limit Situation Made Us All More Philosophical". In: Mossleh, P. ed. 2022. *Corona Phenomenon: Philosophical and Political Questions*. Leiden and Boston: Brill.

Hahn, Edward. 1926. *Der Staat, ein Lebenwesen*. Munich: Dt. Volksverlag.

Hardt, Michael and Antonio Negri. 2000. *Empire*. Cambridge, Mass.: Harvard University Press.

Hardt, Michael and Antonio Negri. 2004. *Multitude: War and Democracy in the Age of Empire*. New York: The Penguin Press.

Hardt, Michael and Antonio Negri. 2009. *Commonwealth*. Cambridge, Mass. Harvard University Press.

Jaspers, Karl. 1954 [2003]. *Way to Wisdom: An Introduction to Philosophy*, second edition, translated by R. Manheim. New Haven and London: Yale University Press.

Kjellén, Rudolf. 1920. *Grundriss zu einem System der Politik*. Leipzig: Rudolf Leipzig Hirzel.

Latour, Bruno. 2018. *Down to Earth: Politics in the New Climatic Regime*, translated by CatherinePorter, Cambridge: Polity Press.

Latour, Bruno. 2021a. *After Lockdown. A Metamorphosis*, translated by J. Rose. Cambridge: Polity Press.

Latour, Bruno. 2021b. "Is This a Dress Rehearsal?", *Critical Inquiry*, 47: S2.

Latour, Bruno and Nikolaj Schultz. 2022. *On the Emergence of an Ecological Class: A Memo*, translated by Julie Rose. Cambridge: Polity.

Lemke, Thomas. 2011. *Biopolitics: An Advanced Introduction*, translated by Eric Frederick Trump. New York: New York University Press.

Massumi, Brian. 2015. *Ontopower: War, Powers, and the State of Perception*. Durham and London: Duke University Press.

Morens, David M., Peter Daszak, Howard Markel, and Jeffrey K. Taubenberger. 2020. "Pandemic COVID-19 Joins History's Pandemic Legion", *mBio*, vol. 11, issue 3, https://doi.org/10.1128/mbio.00812-20. Accessed 23 February 2024.

Morin, Edgar. 1969. *Introduction à une politique de l'homme*. Paris: Éditions du Seuil.

Nancy, Jean-Luc. 2022. *An All-Too-Human Virus*, translated by Cory Stockwell, Sarah Clift and David Fernbach, Cambridge: Polity.

Negri, Antonio. 2008. "The Labor of the Multitude and the Fabric of Biopolitics", translated by Sara Mayo, Peter Graefe and Mark Coté. Ed. Mark Coté. *Mediations*, 23 (2): 8–25.

Negri, Antonio. 2013. *Spinoza for Our Time: Politics and Postmodernity*, translated by William McCuaig. New York: Columbia University Press.

Povinelli, Elizabeth A. 2016. *Geontologies: A Requiem to Late Liberalism*. Durham, London: Duke University Press.

Prozorov, Sergei. 2022. "Lessons from the Pandemic: Biopower, Politics and Reality", *Athena: filosofijos studijos*, eds. Denis Petrina and Audronė Žukauskaitė, No. 17, pp. 16–26.

Roberts, Morley. 1938. *Bio-politics: An Essay in the Physiology, Pathology and Politics of the Social and Somatic Organism*. London: Dent.

Starobinski, Aroon. 1960. *La biopolitique: Essai d'interprétation de l'histoire de l'humanité et des civilisations*. Geneva: Imprimerie des Arts.

Uexküll, Jakob von. 1920. *Staatsbiologie: Anatomie, Physiologie, Pathologie des Staates*. Berlin: Verlag von Gebrüder Paetel.

Virno, Paolo. 2004. *A Grammar of the Multitude: For an Analysis of Contemporary Forms of Life*, translated by Isabella Bertoletti, James Cascaito, Andrea Casson. Semiotext(e).

Yusoff, Kathryn. 2018. *A Billion Black Anthropocenes Or None*. Minneapolis: Minnesota University Press.

Žižek Slavoj. 2020. *Pandemic: COVID-19 Shakes the World*, Cambridge: Polity.

Žižek Slavoj. 2021. *Pandemic 2: Chronicles of a Time Lost*, Cambridge: Polity.

Žukauskaitė, Audronė, Wilmer, S. E. 2016. "Introduction", in *Resisting Biopolitics: Philosophical, Political and Performative Strategies*, eds. S. E. Wilmer and Audronė Žukauskaitė, New York, London: Routledge, pp. 1–18.

PART 1

Biopolitics and Pandemic: Vulnerability, Deprivation, Dispossession

CHAPTER 1

Philosophy as Immunity and Contagion

J. D. Mininger

Abstract

This text considers if and how the experience of the COVID-19 pandemic produced a greater proclivity towards philosophy and philosophical reflection. By way of reflecting on these questions, the chapter considers the propriety and efficacy of understanding philosophy through the health-related guiding metaphors of immunity and contagion – ubiquitous terms during the pandemic. The chapter deploys Karl Jaspers' concept of a "limit situation" to consider these matters and analyzes Plato's famous account of the death of Socrates as a foundational historical and conceptual moment for philosophy considered through the lens of immunity and contagion.

Keywords

COVID-19 – philosophy – immunity – contagion – Socrates

1 The Pandemic, Philosophy, and *Grenzsituationen*

The COVID-19 pandemic was many things – but was it a catalyst for philosophy? Unquestionably, the pandemic experience has motivated academic philosophers to produce commentary on the problems, novel circumstances, stresses, fears, and lessons from the pandemic. Some academic projects, such as this very volume, seek to theorize the pandemic circumstances and events themselves and, at the same time, use the pandemic as a convenient example for explaining, supporting, or challenging already established concepts, interpretations, and frameworks. The bibliography of works in which the COVID-19 pandemic is an object of inquiry or key thematic point of content will, no doubt, continue to grow – and rightly so. However, the opening question asks not merely about academic formats of philosophical productivity, but also about whether the pandemic experience compelled people of all sorts to philosophize. If so, which people (excluding academics)? People who identify as philosophers, or identify as philosophically minded, or enjoy philoso-

 | DOI:10.1163/9789004748187_003

phizing among friends, who would write or think or speak or initiate more philosophy? Non-philosophers who learned about philosophy, inspired by the circumstances of the pandemic? Did the pandemic stimulate the creation of new concepts or the testing of new philosophical truth claims? Did the pandemic circumstances motivate a sudden greater interest in finding renewed relevance in older philosophical texts and ideas? I have neither properly academic nor appropriately philosophical answers to these detailed sub-questions, but the original question can be productively reframed in light of this proliferation of follow-up queries. The real stakes of the question are not so much whether the COVID-19 pandemic was a source for philosophizing – because experience(s) of any sort can elicit philosophically considered responses. Instead, the importance of the question lies in whether the pandemic amplified, accelerated, intensified, or in some way precipitated more philosophizing – whether about the pandemic or anything else.

In his 2022 article, "How a Limit Situation Made Us All More Philosophical," which belongs to one of the first volumes of academic philosophy to be published on the topic of the pandemic, *Corona Phenomenon: Philosophical and Political Questions* (Mossleh 2022), Jean Grondin makes his case for how the pandemic inspired people to think philosophically. He begins by asserting that the pandemic circumstances radically changed most people's expectations of some of the most basic routines of life. Specifically, he notes the requirement to stay home and the related prohibition of meeting with people in a typical way that most would simply take for granted, such as meeting wherever, whenever, without a required medical mask, etc. His point is a simple but profound one: these radical lifestyle changes caused by the COVID-19 pandemic forced many (if not most) people to more emphatically consider what basic rights and opportunities they expect of their lives and, upon that basis, to identify what is most important to them.

Grondin proclaims: "The Corona pandemic reminded us of the forgotten fragility of human life. Forcing us to stay at home as much as possible, to work, to teach, and to learn from home, brought about a more reflective attitude toward life and a reassessing of our priorities. We all became more philosophical" (2022: 32). His point about a forced change in lifestyle leading to greater reflection about priorities is undoubtedly true as a typical and common experience. As the object and insight of those reflections, surely, the reminder that illness and death are potentially always nearer than what we imagine during the oblivion of happiness, ignorance, and routine, is also true. Interestingly, Grondin does not mention another of the most typical pandemic insights, namely, the extraordinary degree of connectedness that people – and planetary life in general – share, which both the spread of the virus and the myriad responses to it across the globe demonstrated over and over again. Why does Grondin elide this second thesis point? He is surely well aware of it, thoughtful philosopher that he is. Major philosophical statements have been penned about this exact revelation regarding connectedness, including in this very volume. It is less important whether Grondin erases, forgets, misses, or ignores; rather, the key point is what he stakes the source of philosophizing on, namely, "the forgotten fragility of human life" (2022: 32). By confronting the thought of death and the concomitant preciousness of life, Grondin suggests that "we all became more philosophical" (2022: 32). But is he correct about this statement?

The COVID-19 pandemic likely prompted many individuals worldwide to contemplate various existential questions and philosophical concepts, whether they recognized their thinking as "philosophical" or not. Due to the tragic loss of loved ones, their own illness, or just the sheer reported numbers of people affected by the virus, many probably woke up to their own vulnerability and fragility. But there are many other potentially equally powerful sources for existential questioning that the pandemic produced – why does Grondin focus only on suffering and death? For example, lockdowns and social distancing measures forced many people into isolation and solitude, providing ample time for introspection. At the end of his article, Grondin reveals his hope that "when this crisis is over, something of this philosophical, monastical, and meditative life might survive, so that we might become less blinded by the frenzied pace of our modern lives and its electronic mirages" (2022: 35). Grondin claims philosophy to be an antidote to certain trends of modern life that he (no doubt in many ways correctly) views as obstacles to critical thinking and human flourishing. This draws an inherent link between philosophical reflection and a secluded, solitary lifestyle. As he notes, while potentially "exasperating, excruciating even, for many, but monastic life can be conducive to philosophy" (Grondin 2022: 35). This suggests that while philosophy does not require a reclusive or withdrawn lifestyle, philosophy is associated inherently with meditation and contemplation.

Before returning to this point for greater scrutiny, there are still other notable sources for philosophizing generated by the pandemic context. The feelings of uncertainty and instability that many felt when the pandemic disrupted their lives in profound ways led some to grapple with questions about the nature of change, impermanence, and resilience, and equally in relation to their own fragility. The pandemic raised ethical dilemmas regarding issues such as resource allocation, healthcare prioritization, and individual responsibilities to society. Together with the aforementioned interconnectedness of the global community and the collective vulnerability of humanity, this awareness may have prompted reflection on concepts of global citizenship, empathy, and the ethical implications of our actions on both individual and global scales. Perhaps even without initial insight into life's fragility, seeking consolation in the face of experiences of fear, sadness, and despair is sufficient to promote philosophizing. In the face of adversity, individuals often turn to philosophy as a kind of spirituality in the hope of finding meaning, hope, and resilience. Many philosophical traditions offer various perspectives on finding meaning and purpose in life, which can provide solace and guidance during challenging times. But whether and how philosophy is, can be, or even should be a kind of (a practice of) spirituality must also be briefly shelved to responsibly attend to the concept Grondin offers as a clarifying lens that aligns all of these possible sources for philosophizing into a common legible image.

Grondin proposes Karl Jaspers' construct of a *Grenzsituation* – limit situation – as a concept capable of unifying and explaining how the abrupt lifestyle changes brought about by the pandemic led to philosophizing: "Limit situations make us more philosophical and certainly more aware of our basic conditions of finite and vulnerable beings" (2022: 35). Grondin explains: "For Jaspers, the basic limit situations were those of death, suffering, tragedy, despair, and defeat, experiences that confront life with its inescapable frailty, thus revealing existence to itself. This pandemic is certainly such a limit situation. It puts things into perspective, relativizing many of the petty concerns of our pre-COVID routine" (2022: 34). Jaspers theorizes the *Grenzsituation* (among other places in his writings) in *Way to Wisdom: An Introduction to Philosophy*, in a section of the book, in which he interrogates key sources of philosophizing. He distinguishes between the beginning(s) of philosophy and sources of philosophy, i.e., what instigates philosophical thinking and action: "The history of philosophy as methodical thinking began twenty-five hundred years ago, but as mythical thought much earlier. The beginning, however, is something quite different from the source. The beginning is historical, and provides those who follow with a mounting accumulation of insights. But it is always from the source that the impulsion to philosophize springs" (Jaspers 1954 [2003]: 15). Jaspers enumerates these key sources as a triad: wonder, doubt, and self-awareness. Wonderment is the ultimate well-spring of inquiry. Doubt sharpens and actively validates existing and emerging knowledge. Self-awareness is the result of self-inquiry, which arises out of the ignorance we typically maintain with regard to the truths of our immediate circumstances due to routine and petty day-to-day concerns.

Jaspers contends that this third source (self-awareness) ushers from a context foundational to our human existence: "We are always in situations. Situations change, opportunities arise. If they are missed they never return. I myself can work to change the situation. But there are situations which remain essentially the same even if their momentary aspect changes and their shattering force is obscured: I must die, I must suffer, I must struggle, I am subject to chance, I involve myself inexorably in guilt. We call these fundamental situations of our existence ultimate situations" (1954 [2003]: 19–20). Ralph Manheim here translates *Grenzsituation* as "ultimate situation," in contrast to Grondin's translation choice of "limit situation," a translation choice shared by many who write on Jaspers. "Limit situation" is a more literal translation of the German *Grenzsituation*. One might say of this liminal situation that it is not merely a limit concept but also a *limiting* experience. "Limit situation" suggests an experience constituted by – and perhaps equally constitutive of – a border or a borderline experience. The *Grenzsituation*, therefore, as Jaspers wields it in this context, refers to an experience in which one is pulled in two directions at once, marked by a (border)line – a meridian – between what we can control and what we cannot. After all, one can only have control if it is possible also not to have control. Thus, while the experience that Jaspers describes includes becoming (self-)aware of weakness and helplessness (Jaspers 1954 [2003]: 19), at the same time, its Janus-faced figuration includes the potential for domination and mastery. This meridian experience is reminiscent of psychoanalyst Jacques Lacan's renowned theory of the foundations of self-identification and self-representation in what he called the mirror stage, in which anticipated self-mastery becomes the motor of desire that fundamentally drives the subject (Lacan 2006). Lacan, however, despite the structural parallels to some aspects of Jaspers' concept of the *Grenzsituation*, does not attend to the affective context (such as death and suffering) in the same way as Jaspers the existentialist, with perhaps the exception of guilt.

For Grondin's deployment of Jaspers' concept, Manheim's translation choice of "ultimate situation" opens an important horizon of understanding. "Ultimate" resonates much better, for example, with Immanuel Kant's category of the sublime, as elucidated in the first section, second book of *The Power of the Critique of Judgment*, titled "Analytic of the Sublime" (2000: 128–159). For Kant, the sublime is an experience of the subject – not a trait or condition of an object – that uncannily balances a certain kind of pleasure in noting one's own safety in the face of a felt danger with a heightened sense of helplessness attendant to that same danger. Kant understands the importance of the sublime as providing a description and an explanation of how individuals move from empirical thoughts of danger and refuge to considerations about what unconditional security might look like in the face of simply existing in the world (as such). For Kant, it is the moral "I" that can guarantee this unconditional refuge. But for the context at hand the importance of the connection between Jaspers' *Grenzsituation* and Kant's theory of the sublime is that, in similar ways, both refer to borderline experiences in which what may be controlled and what may not be controlled are ultimately at stake. Beginning with Kierkegaard and developed emphatically by Heidegger, this liminal experience was otherwise named as the distinction between fear and anxiety. In *A Grammar of the Multitude*, Paulo Virno provides the following description of this context:

> The Kantian distinction between the two types of risk and security is drawn out in the distinction, traced by Heidegger, between fear and anguish. Fear refers to a very specific fact, to the familiar snowslide or to the loss of one's job; anguish, instead, has no clear cause which sparks it off. In the pages of Heidegger's *Being and Time* [...] anguish is provoked purely and simply by our being exposed to the world, by the uncertainty and indecision with which our relation to this world manifests itself. Fear is always circumscribed and nameable; anguish is ubiquitous, not connected to distinctive causes; it can survive in any given moment or situation.
>
> 2004: 33

The *Grenzsituation* to which Jaspers refers is the experience of anxiety, in which a fundamental, ultimate experience arises because the unique nature (among all affects) of the object of that anxiety is precisely to be objectless. For Jaspers, the uniqueness of an "ultimate situation" is that the inescapable realities are the points of the ultimately unknown, most notably, death (and fragility of life); or, for Heidegger, in the more ontological and conceptual idiom, the Nothing. The "ultimate" quality of the situation, therefore, refers to circumstances in which (supposedly) unavoidable truths are immutable and insurmountable; they cannot be controlled and ultimately mastered; and they certainly cannot be transcended. They can only be recognized and acknowledged for their being thusly.

The crucial follow-up question is: how do we understand ourselves in the transition from self-inquiry to self-awareness through the experience of what Jaspers calls a *Grenzsituation*, and with which Grondin labels the pandemic? What do we learn about ourselves in this process? After all, one of Western philosophy's oldest mottos refers precisely to this: know thyself! Grondin explains that "we learn through experiences that call into question our expectations because they force us to rethink our ways and become more reflective, more philosophical about things" (2022: 34–35). For example, there is a great distinction between, on one hand, acknowledging the unavoidable fact of death by lament and despair about one's fate and, on the other hand, greeting the fact of mortality with the same content of perception but with a different quality of perceiving, such that, without denying or ignoring it, this thought of death no longer troubles one's appreciation of the present. Is this latter procedure what is meant by being "more philosophical about things?" (Grondin 2022: 35). Assuming so, Grondin's initial claim seems accurate: indubitably, the pandemic created "ultimate situations" for many people, in which more unusual intensities of self-reflection expressed potentially new insights about themselves and their own awareness of themselves, their identities, and their very existence.

I share Grondin's immediate and subsequent question: "what is it to become more *philosophical*?" (2022, 35 [emphasis in the original]) Ultimately, an answer to this question lies hidden and dispersed in the manifold interstices of answers to the questions: what does it mean to do philosophy, to practice philosophical thinking, to be a philosopher, to express oneself philosophically, and to interact with others in a philosophical mode of engagement and collaboration? For this reason, the answer can probably only ever be tentative and preliminary. It should be expressed in the contours of immanent causality: philosophy exists only in its effects, that is, (a) philosophy is an effect of its own effects (cf. Kordela 2007). Sounding not unlike Gilles Deleuze, a philosopher from which he is otherwise decidedly dissimilar, Karl Jaspers explains this problem of defining philosophy and philosophizing in a way that understands philosophy as an act of singularities on a lived plane of immanence:

> There is nothing above or beside philosophy. It cannot be derived from something else. Every philosophy defines itself by its realization. We can determine the nature of philosophy only by actually experiencing it. Philosophy then becomes the realization of the living idea and the reflection upon this idea, action and discourse on action in one. Only by thus experiencing philosophy for ourselves can we understand previously formulated philosophical thought.
>
> 1954 [2003]: 13

We know we have philosophized, in the sense of naming it as such, only retroactively, only in a moment of reflection. Philosophy, therefore, is singular in its lived contextual coordinates and irreducibly multiple, mutable, even fungible, as "previously formulated philosophical thought" (Jaspers 1954 [2003]: 13).

Grondin's answer to his own question contains none of this nuance; however, it does faithfully attend to the specific pandemic context within which his philosophizing emerges in this instance. He writes:

> What does it mean to become more *philosophical*? It does not mean that we start to study philosophy or to read difficult books of philosophy. Fundamentally, it means that we learn to display calm, wisdom, and serenity in the presence of adversity. Limit situations make us more philosophical and certainly more aware of our basic condition of finite and vulnerable beings, which we tend to forget when the breakneck pace of *normal* life takes hold of us.
>
> 2022: 35, emphases in the original

Grondin describes his definition of philosophizing in and for this specific context using coordinates that happen to align with how Spinoza describes the relation(s) of bodies at the most fundamental level(s): "motion and rest, speed and slowness" (Spinoza 2000: 126). Grondin explains philosophizing here as insight won through experience (i.e., wisdom) expressed or presented in a mode and milieu of tranquility – despite adverse conditions. In the context of this essay, "adversity" clearly refers to a confrontation with a thought that he names in his opening sentence: "the forgotten fragility of human life" (2022: 32). As the pandemic reminded people of the (literally) breathtaking proximity of death in ways more frequent and intense than in earlier "normal" pre-pandemic life, Grondin sees philosophy as a means whereby we remain calm and composed – untroubled – in the experience of this "ultimate situation." For Grondin, there is a (high) speed to "normal life," and he poses philosophizing as a vastly decelerated speed. Where there is agitation due to the dread and danger attendant to an "ultimate situation," so that (supposedly) philosophy supplies the tools for learning how to proceed slowly, smoothly, and peacefully.

There is nothing novel in positioning philosophy within this ethological dichotomy of "motion and rest, speed and slowness" as the privileged coordinate point(s) of slowness and rest. Notably, this cliché abounds in Western philosophy textbooks when describing variations of rationalism from Stoicism to the present. This formula of philosophy's tranquility in addressing adversity is often applied to rationalism and the possibility of reason to surmount and, at times, fully transcend the emotions. This "mind over matter" approach often applies the superiority of the mind over the body, just as the metaphorical coordinates of the varying intensities of temperature (which themselves are ultimately extrapolations of the fundamental matrix of motion and rest, speed and slowness) – reason as cool and emotion as hot – mark innumerable accounts of philosophy's fundamental structures.

Isaac Bashevis Singer's short story "The Spinoza of Market Street" provides a narrative account of this clichéd approach. The short story tells the tale of an aging man, Dr. Fischelson, who has dedicated his life to studying Spinoza's *Ethics*, upon whose basis he has tried consistently to root out the pleasures of the moment as he lives in pursuit of what he believes Spinoza's philosophy teaches about the freeing and the perfection of the mind. By the time of his old age he has had what we are to understand is, by most standards, a dull, lonely, and difficult life, and his attempt to live out Spinoza's philosophy is the one significant remedy to his struggles, which he has applied – until in the twilight of his life he marries the spinster next door and on their wedding night feels "powers long dormant awakened in him" (Singer 2004: 92). While clearly, the story satirizes the quasi-monastic, rationalist, mind-over-matter interpretation of Spinoza's philosophy that the character reveres, the story ends with a poignant line that avails itself of potentially two contradictory readings of the entire story's dramatization of Spinoza's philosophy: "Divine Spinoza, forgive me. I have become a fool" (Singer 2004: 93). Genevieve Lloyd explains the ending's dramatic ambiguity in the following way:

> Is it his lapse into the "pleasure of the moment" or his former illusion that, "seen from above", that lapse matters, that we are supposed to see as the folly for which he asks Spinoza's forgiveness? It is possible to read this ironic tale as satirizing a life led in accordance with Spinoza's philosophy. It is also possible to read it as a progress to a richer understanding of that philosophy – as the story of a movement from a self-centered preoccupation with the pursuit of a sterile version of reason to a richer appreciation of what is really involved in perceiving the world and its transitory pleasure *sub specie aeternitatis.*
>
> 1996: 59–60

The story reinforces the clichés of the detached, calm philosopher by seeming to criticize and poke fun at Dr. Fischelson's understanding of and approach to Spinoza – here understood to be a dedicated, perhaps even zealous rationalist. In the end, the man asks Spinoza's forgiveness because he feels that by giving in to the seductions of desires of the flesh and emotional connectedness to others, he has betrayed the philosophy's foundations rooted in detached, cool, and serene reflection. As Lloyd points out, the story suggests that there may be more complex interpretations that compel further consideration. But the story also points to the potential danger inherent in manifesting that clichéd version of philosophy: namely, that pleasure, meaning, and even redemption may be obscured by the very act – philosophizing – that otherwise promises them.

Gilles Deleuze and Felix Guattari indicate a similar dynamic when they (partially) define philosophy in the introduction to their powerful *What Is Philosophy?* as the discipline and act of creating concepts (1994). Specifically, they oppose the passé image of philosophy as rationalist and detached by suggesting what philosophy is not, namely, contemplation, reflection, and communication (Deleuze and Guattari 1994: 6). They do not suggest that these three dimensions are excluded from the execution of what might be called philosophizing, but none of the three belong to or express the essence of philosophy as creating concepts. This definition does not have to be set at odds with Grondin's claim to becoming more philosophical due to the pandemic context. This volume's contribution to rethinking biopolitics in the wake of the pandemic expresses the spirit of Deleuze and Guattari's definition of philosophy as the creation of concepts. However, their understanding of what constitutes and animates philosophy does not align well with the understanding of philosophy as merely detached, calm reflections in the face of anxiety and/of "ultimate situations."

In addition to Grondin's own question – "what is it to become more *philosophical*?" – the inquiry can be productively pressed a step further: what is it to become *more* philosophical? In terms borrowed from pandemic vocabulary and in line with the themes of this volume, we might say that Grondin's characterization of philosophizing suggests that being "philosophical" provides *immunity* against the *contagion* of "situations which remain essentially the same even if their momentary aspect changes and their shattering force is obscured: I must die, I must suffer, I must struggle, I am subject to chance, I involve myself inexorably in guilt. We call these fundamental situations of our existence ultimate situations" (Jaspers 1954 [2003]: 19–20). How much philosophizing is needed to inoculate one against the workings of these ultimately unavoidable infections?

Just as there is nothing novel in positioning philosophy as slowness and calm, to posit philosophy as a healing agent is equally unoriginal, though not for that reason unproductive or without benefit. The tradition of Western philosophy, from its very inception, has positioned itself as an antidote to various poisons, whether those be the dangers of falsehood, spiritual degradation, suffering, etc. Immunity and contagion are fundamental idioms for understanding the purpose(s) of philosophy. The pandemic's literal–biological plague of contagion, and our becoming more philosophical as a search for and practice of immunity, takes us back to the place where arguably the Western philosophical tradition was founded – but therefore to a beginning that is the narration of an ending: the story of Socrates' death.

2 Socrates, Philosophy, and Immunity

Michel Foucault's 1983–1984 lectures at the *Collège de France*, titled *The Courage of Truth* (2011), provide a rich, learned, cogent, and compelling philosophical narrative about philosophy's roots as an act and practice of (self-)immunization. This story follows the conceptual protagonist "Truth" from its initial situation as truth-telling through a process of distillation and separation from other modes of truth-telling. In particular, Foucault refines it from political veridiction to an ethical form of parrhesia concerned with awakening others to care for themselves. Foucault reconstructs the Greek concept of *parrhesia* – frank speech, truth-telling without decoration, veridiction in its plain, "raw" form – and assimilates discourse on ancient Cynicism and its transhistorical perseverance beyond the ancient tradition through such iterations as Christian asceticism, political revolutionary subjectivity of the nineteenth century, and the modern art and artists of the twentieth century. Eventually, as a narrative, Foucault takes Truth across a dénouement in which truth-telling effectively becomes a kind of truth-living, a mode of veridiction concerned more with life (*bios*) than with the soul (for instance), and more focused on a testing of life and rendering account of oneself not as an essence or singular form but as an adequate relation between one's self and the logos one proclaims. Foucault initially mines the concept of ethical parrhesia from Plato's Socrates in the *Apology* and draws especially from the *Laches*. But he eventually locates its most characteristic practice in the example of the Cynics, in which Foucault sees a major alternative to Platonism. But even if "Truth" (as ethical parrhesia) is the conceptual protagonist of the plotline that Foucault endeavors to unveil slowly over the course of his lectures, he still manifests this in a conceptual persona: Socrates.

The stakes of this narration are higher than just Socrates' story of how philosophy's parrhesia immunized him from false discourses. Foucault himself, as a narrator–lecturer, quietly doubles Socrates' own story by encouraging others to care for themselves as he nears his own death. In compelling respects, these lectures are a mimetic response to his own study of Socrates' death cycle. Foucault's final lectures constitute a double articulation: a discourse of and about parrhesia. To "read" the parrhesiacal performance that doubles the teacherly presentation, we must access both the context and genesis of the lecture text, as well as the seemingly inconsequential opening comments and closing remarks that book-end his lecture series. These lectures were Foucault's last. He had been battling illness over the winter of 1983–84, and his lectures began three weeks late due to severe ill health. He was treated in a Paris hospital regularly during March – the lectures occurred once a week from February 1 to March 28 – and two-and-a-half months later, in June, Foucault died. He certainly knew his health was poor, and he surely suspected that it was HIV-AIDS from which he was dying, though accounts suggest Foucault did not inquire about these matters with the doctors, asking only about how much time they thought he had. These lectures are not a form of last testament; but, without question, these lectures proceed within a horizon shadowed by impending death, including the thought and anticipation of death – a *Grenz-situation*, indeed.

Consider the opening words of the lectures, which the volume editors assume are so relatively insignificant that they are not placed in the main body of the text as the opening of the lectures but are provided only in tiny footnote-sized font at the bottom of the page: "I was not able to start my lectures as usual at the beginning of January. I was ill, really ill. There were rumors saying that changing the dates was a way for me to get rid of some of my auditors. Not at all, I was really ill" (Foucault 2011: 1). With the asterisk of Foucault's death several months later retroactively looming over a reading of the text like a dark cloud or omen, the lectures accept an additional untimely hue – late lectures under the shadow of impending death. Even his final spoken words on the last lecture day ring of lateness, pregnant with the event of death to come: "There you are, listen, I had things to say to you about the general framework of these analyses. But, well, it is too late. So, thank you" (Foucault 2011: 338). One gets the sense that perhaps it is always too late: for a truth that must be lived, for a truth that requires an essential position of otherness, for a truth that is never the same, to speak it and to require its form as logos is to assign it always already to a situation in which it will always come too late because it can only ever arrive untimely, too late: or never at all.

With these bookends, Foucault's lecture text binds together work and life in a mutually determining package: the thought of death implicates both subject and object, philosopher and concept, and artist and artwork. In so doing, it raises the stakes and the question of if and how truth may be communicated more transparently or directly through an individual style or mode. But before problematizing this timely lateness, let us note the crucial choice of texts by which Foucault molds his concept of ethical parrhesia: Socrates' death cycle – specifically, the *Apology* and the *Phaedo*. These are not merely texts about lateness and death – these are founding texts of Western philosophy. In fact, it will be Foucault's claim that "Socrates' death founds philosophy, in the reality of Greek thought and therefore in Western history, as a form of veridiction which is not that of prophecy, or wisdom, or tekhne; a form of veridiction peculiar precisely to philosophical discourse, and the courage of which must be exercised until death as a test of the soul which cannot take place on the political platform" (2011: 114). The founding of philosophy as a form of parrhesia was an untimely act practiced towards life in the form of care, predicated upon a peculiar relation to death in the form of the courage to ignore death in favor of the constant mission of encouraging others to care for themselves. In the *Apology*, Foucault concentrates his commentary on Socrates' relation to the risk of death attached to his truth-telling. In the *Phaedo*, he looks to Socrates' final words prior to dying, interpreting them as a kind of last testament in which parrhesia as the practice of urging others to care for themselves becomes the mission of philosophy.

From what Foucault extracts from Plato's *Apology*, he focuses on the matter of how Socrates negotiated the risks run by his parrhesia. The seeming conundrum is that throughout the text, Socrates says that he did not and does not fear death; yet if he does not fear death, "how is it that in this defense he says: I have not engaged in politics because if I had done so I would be dead?" (Foucault 2011: 80). The initial animating question is why Socrates does not tell the truth politically, in a political way? Why does he not defend himself in an overtly political manner? Does he abstain from politics out of fear of death? Clearly, Socrates' veridiction bears with it the possible risk of death. Foucault's explanation is: Socrates does not avoid politics for fear of death. What Foucault admits is that "he did abstain from politics because of these dangers, not out of fear of death, but because if he had got involved in politics he would be dead and, being dead, he would have been unable – as he says in the text – to be useful to himself and to the Athenians" (2011: 80). So, Socrates does avoid death, not because it is evil, painful, or scary, but because it would prevent him from being able to effect the positive change he feels called to achieve. Death is an inconvenience that Socrates avoids in order to fulfill his philosophical mission. In the spirit of care of the self, Socrates takes care of himself so as to be able to fulfill his mission of encouraging others to care for themselves. He is courageous in sticking to this mission of philosophy, that is, ethical truth-telling. This ethical parrhesia unfolds very differently from political parrhesia, where truth is delivered courageously, but aimed at telling "an Assembly or a tyrant who does not want to hear it" what to do (Foucault 2011: 87). By telling the truth otherwise than strictly politically, Socrates manages to be useful to the city, to care for the demos, and to urge others to attend to their own needs. Socrates satisfied the ideals of political action and veridiction precisely by abandoning his commitment to political veridiction. Socrates manages to achieve politics in his very rejection of politics, thanks to his peculiar relationship to death – or, in reference to Jaspers' concept, thanks to his singular response to this *Grenzsituation*.

Phaedo is another text situated under the shadow of death. This time Foucault's point of emphasis is on the "strange banality" and largely "unexplained" qualities of Socrates' reported last words, to which Foucault will assign enormous value, in contradistinction to a long-standing traditional interpretation (2011: 96). Plato's *Phaedo* reports Socrates' last words to be: "Crito, we owe a cock to Asclepius. Pay my debt, don't forget" (quoted in Foucault 2011: 96). Asclepius is the god whose one relation to humans is to cure them. Thus, the question arises: how did Socrates suffer such that he needed to be cured, and for which cure does Socrates owe a rooster to Asclepius as a debt of gratitude? The traditional interpretation is that Socrates thanks Asclepius (i.e., owes the debt of sacrificing a rooster) because death will cure him of the disease of life. As Foucault points out, even Nietzsche, though slightly skeptical, still ultimately subscribes to this explanation that Socrates essentially tells Crito that life is a disease, even if that contradicts how Socrates had addressed himself to life up until this point of his very final words. One suspects a strong influence of the Christian tradition here in the enduring traditional interpretation of Socrates' last words, in the form of the flesh as sinful and life as a disease that death and salvation can cure.

But if the disease of life is not that which is cured, what is this cure? What is this activity by which Socrates and his friends have been cured? According to Foucault, the activity that effects the cure is *epimeleia* – care. Initially, it is a concern of the gods for men, upon which the care of self and others is based. What is the disease that is cured if life is not itself the disease? That seems entirely inconsistent with Socrates' approach to philosophical life, which was "the pure life, the life untroubled by any passion, any desire, any unrestrained appetite, and false opinion" (Foucault 2011: 100–1). The action of this *epimeleia* (care) is truth. The truth, in determining what is just and unjust, is what must lead us to care not about opinions but about those people and actions and ideas that lead us to truth. It is philosophy – parrhesia – that, to the end, to death, in perpetual "lateness," cures Socrates of the disease of prejudice, false opinions, and false discourse. By requesting to sacrifice a cock to Asclepius, Socrates thanks the gods for philosophy and the truth-telling that kept him "healthy" to the end. Foucault explains:

> Caring for someone, looking after a flock, taking care of one's family, or, as is often found with regard to physicians, caring for a patient, are all called "epimeleisthai." The curing that Socrates speaks about here is part of all those activities by which one cares for someone, takes care of him if he is ill, sees to his diet so that he does not fall ill, prescribes the food he must eat or the exercises he must perform, and it is also part of those

> activities by which one points out to him the actions he should perform and those he should avoid, by which one helps him to discover the true opinions he should follow and the false opinions he should guard against, it is that activity by which one nourishes him with true discourse.
>
> 2011: 110

Thus, Socrates' mission concerning the care of the self leads to his death, and it is in his death that he can bear this gift along to others, both in wishing that humans take care of themselves and referring to the gods' care for humans so that they care for themselves. This version of philosophy rooted in ethical parrhesia grounds philosophy and, through the figure of Socrates, founds the philosophical tradition as an immunization.

3 Philosophy, Immunity, and Contagion

The story of Socrates being immunized by his philosophical activity, which protected him from the contagious diseases of prejudice and false discourses up until his death, fits nicely as a support and decoration for Grondin's claim that the pandemic made us more philosophical. Grondin paints a relatively (philosophically) pretty picture of the pandemic scene. He decorates it as a redemptive prospect, in which philosophical reflection and self-inquiry arise from suffering and the "limit situation" confrontations. His claim suggests that more people questioned the purpose of their existence; more dove deep into self-interrogation; and more stared suffering and even death in the face and, in the enforced monastic setting of lockdown, serenely philosophized in the slow pace and serene setting of their homes. But for this philosophizing to enact its inoculating function and not merely be the hollow shell of a seemingly philosophical practice, or what in the metaphor here we should call a "placebo effect," the philosophizing must have some potency.

Philosophy's immunity-granting properties may be less accessible than Grondin's pretty picture presents. For many people, knowing oneself is assumed to be a challenging but achievable goal because of our typical understanding of the relationship between knowledge and truth. At least in its original context, philosophy's foundational act – the Delphic precept to "know yourself" – was more than merely an accumulation of the knowledge (i.e., information) that we have and know and believe about ourselves.

In his 1981–1982 lectures, *The Hermeneutics of the Subject*, Foucault argues that in the course of Western thought and education – at the moment of the Cartesian intervention – the maxim "know yourself" became delinked from the imperative to care for yourself, which Foucault contends was always implied in the original Hellenistic and Roman understanding. Foucault argues that modernity's relation to truth "begins when knowledge itself and knowledge alone gives access to the truth" (Foucault 2005: 17). The result for modern science and modern knowledge is that:

> the subject's being is not put in question by the necessity of having access to truth … Knowledge will simply open out onto the indefinite dimension of progress, the end of which is unknown and the advantage of which will only ever be realized in the course of history by the institutional accumulation of bodies of knowledge, or the psychological or social benefits to be had from having discovered the truth after having taken such pains to do so.
>
> FOUCAULT 2005: 18–19

As subjects, we are essentially no longer at stake in our own knowledge if "know yourself" excludes the foundation practice of "care of the self." With this approach to self-knowing as our philosophizing, the "limit situations" described by Jaspers will hardly be responsibly processed and addressed, let alone properly acknowledged. The lack of control that Jaspers suggests belongs to an ultimate situation as exactly the borderline element that motivates the fundamental anxiety emanating from the danger at hand is effectively avoided if nothing of ourselves is risked in the process of accessing truth – whether about ourselves or anything else. In short, for knowledge to be something other than a kind of self-fulfilling prophecy, we must risk not knowing how it will all play out on the other side! For access to truth, we must risk ourselves as we currently know ourselves. Philosophy as care of the self, embodied in Socrates, who "knew himself" by "caring for himself," has the power to protect from the contagion and disease of false discourse. But are we moderns now hardwired in such a way that we are prepared to seek access to truth through self-inquiry in the way Socrates "immunized" himself?

I am tempted to suggest that alongside the COVID-19 pandemic, we continue to experience a parallel plague, which aligns all too well with Socrates' fears: the plague of prejudice and false discourse that today goes by the names of disinformation and conspiracy theories. Admittedly, there is much discourse about these poisons, though not enough that is antidotal. But the focus of this text is not so much the disease as the supposed expansion of philosophical remedy. Therefore, I repeat the challenge to Grondin's thesis: did we really immunize ourselves from false discourse by becoming more philosophical during the pandemic?

Philosophizing can immunize, but not merely as a cure for various diseases of discourse and mind. Philosophy is not a simple truth pill. I harbor one great concern about understanding philosophy as inoculation – even when that fundamental metaphor ushers from philosophy's own founder and patron saint, Socrates. Philosophizing can and should only immunize to the degree that it provides immunity against the disease of consolation. Socrates' gratitude for philosophy keeping him "healthy" to the end was not comfort in place of having suffered. His was not Boethius' consolation. Socrates' gratitude was not about helping to put death in its correct and understandable place. One of philosophy's most surprising and important "healing" powers may be to provide immunity against consolation in the form of risk-free access to truth. Philosophy need not make us feel good to work its healing powers. Philosophizing requires risk and, at times, a lack of safety and protection within our thoughts, including where those thoughts might lead. Self-inquiry may not be calm and serene; it might require significant agitation and speed of thought and life.

Philosophy can traffic in happiness; however, happiness is not the goal of philosophy. Equally, happiness is only one of many satisfactory outcomes of meeting a *Grenzsituation* with rigorous philosophical engagement. In its parallel forms as thought and action, philosophy has a Paracelsian sense, namely, that our concepts, insights, and new experiences are a poison with the results based on dosage: it can immunize and heal, or it can also inflict suffering and harm. Philosophy pills worth the name should come with a safety label.

Philosophy can provide and protect the health of the mind and spirit, but health is a relative term. Philosophy's demands might appear as a plague to normal health, such as in the case of what Nietzsche referred to in aphorism #382 of *The Gay Science* as "great health": an intellectual fitness of strength and energy required for as yet unthought thoughts and unrealized creative potentials (Nietzsche 2001: 246). Nietzsche describes the philosophers of the future as requiring "a new health that is stronger, craftier, tougher, holder, and more cheerful than any previous health" (Nietzsche 2001: 246), precisely because seeking out novel concepts and creative approaches requires new sources, pathways, and means. The new health requires change and risk of losing control, not prefigured knowledge and security of consistent control.

What potentiates health in the *Grenzsituation* is precisely the danger to one's health. The shock of difference, of otherness, that confronts us in a *Grenzsituation* can be a poison or antidote, but neither is mere consolation, i.e., the idea of access to truth without the risk of transformation and change. Nietzsche describes the "great health" required of philosophy as precisely this matter of consistent intellectual peril: "anyone who wants to know from the adventures of his own experience how it feels to be the discoverer or conqueror of an ideal, or to be an artist, a saint, a lawmaker, a sage, a pious man, a soothsayer, an old-style divine Ioner – any such person needs one thing above all – the great health, a health that one doesn't only have, but also acquires continually and must acquire because one gives it up again and again, and must give it up!" (Nietzsche 2001: 246). At root, one risks philosophical health at every step because access to truth requires the possibility that what you find is not what you are now.

Philosophers, both uninitiated and long-experienced, young and old, contradict the essence of philosophy by assuming that the health their philosophizing seeks to protect should require their possession of truth. Whether they are motivated to become "more philosophical" by the pandemic or fighting to maintain arbitrary disciplinary territories within outdated and long-stagnant academic sub-fields (the lack of "great health" of which may be marked precisely by the supposed health of an ever-growing bibliography of academic articles), or any other variety and profile, there are always those that immunize themselves with lethal doses of philosophical poison in the form of the assumption that philosophy's baseline for health is possession of truth – in particular in the form of replicable and repeatable knowledge. In such cases, the tropology breaks down because the next requirement would be an immunization against immunizations.

I hope that Jean Grondin is correct in his claim that in the wake of the COVID-19 pandemic, we became more philosophical. But I strongly doubt this is the case. The challenge of philosophy's source of health will never appeal to broad masses; this is precisely why Socrates' mission was to encourage others to know and care for themselves. The reality of philosophy's baseline for health can be found in its famous namesake – the love of wisdom – which refers most emphatically to the *search* for truth rather than any possession of it. In this way, philosophy itself is something of an ultimate, borderline concept, in which the loved object is desired and necessarily always just out of reach. This must surely be what Foucault refers to in the final words of the manuscript of his last lecture, where he had written (but, with uncanny untimeliness, did not even have time to deliver) the sublimely distilled phrases that summarize the stakes of philosophy's own health and purposes: "there is no establishment of the truth without an essential position of otherness; the truth is never the same; there can be truth only in the form of the other world and the other life (l'autre monde et de la vie autre)" (Foucault 2011: 356).

References

Deleuze, G., and Guattari, F. 1994. *What Is Philosophy?* translated by H. Tomlinson and G. Burchell. New York: Columbia University Press.

Foucault, M. 2005. *The Hermeneutics of the Subject: Lectures at the Collège de France 1981–1982*, translated by G. Burchell and edited by F. Gros. New York: Palgrave Macmillan.

Foucault, M. 2011. *The Courage of Truth. The Government of Self and Others II: Lectures at the Collège de France, 1983–1984*, translated by G. Burchell, edited by F. Gros. New York: Palgrave Macmillan.

Grondin, J. 2022. "How a Limit Situation Made Us All More Philosophical". In: Mossleh, P. ed. 2022. *Corona Phenomenon: Philosophical and Political Questions.* Leiden and Boston: Brill.

Jaspers, K. 1954 [2003]. *Way to Wisdom: An Introduction to Philosophy*, second edition, translated by R. Manheim. New Haven and London: Yale University Press.

Kant, I. 2000. *Critique of the Power of Judgment*, edited by P. Guyer and translated by P. Guyer and E. Matthews. Cambridge: Cambridge University Press.

Kordela, K. 2007. *$urplus: Spinoza, Lacan.* Albany: State University of New York Press.

Lacan, J. 2006. The Mirror Stage as Formative of the Function of the I as Revealed at Psychoanalytic Experience. In: B. Fink (Trans.), *Écrits: The First Complete Edition in English.* New York/London: W.W. Norton and Company.

Latour, Bruno. 2018. *Down to Earth: Politics in the New Climatic Regime*, trans. Catherine Porter, Cambridge: Polity Press.

Lloyd, G. 1996. *Spinoza and the Ethics.* Routledge: London.

Mossleh, P. ed. 2022. *Corona Phenomenon: Philosophical and Political Questions.* Leiden and Boston: Brill.

Nietzsche, F. 2001. *The Gay Science*, edited by B. Williams and translated by J. Nauckhoff. Cambridge: Cambridge University Press.

Singer, I.B. 2004. *Complete Stories.* New York: Literary Classics of the United States, Inc.

Spinoza, B. 2000. *Ethics*, edited and translated by G.H.R. Parkinson. Oxford: Oxford University Press.

Virno, P. 2004. *A Grammar of the Multitude. For an Analysis of Contemporary Forms of Life.* Los Angeles: Semiotext(e).

CHAPTER 2

Total Lockdown: the Pandemic and Affective Disorders

Denis Petrina

Abstract

The phrase "total lockdown" in the first part of the title refers to a universal existential condition, which we have experienced during the pandemic and still experience today to some extent, mainly caused by the negation of life as a vital force (*vita activa*). The second part of the title – "The Pandemic and Affective Disorders" – highlights the affective imbalances arising not only at a personal but also at a more universal – social and political – level. This chapter explores what affects, feelings, sensations, and experiences have spread, how we "contract" them, and how (and whether) we deal with them. The research question of the chapter addresses the challenge of verbalizing and signifying affective experiences of the pandemic, which is complicated by the inherent resistance of affect to language. This chapter analyzes the pandemic through the lens of the interplay between the material conditions and outcomes of the pandemic and the discursive formations that both reinforce and are shaped by them. The chapter focuses on the inevitable tension between the hegemonic discourse on/of the pandemic, which encapsulates and homogenizes a wide range of affective responses to the "total lockdown," and the affective drama that is taking place behind the "smokescreen" of this discourse. The chapter considers how to articulate this drama while balancing individual experiences with their universal *commonality*. Ultimately, the chapter examines narratives and techniques that transgress beyond the discourse insensitive to pandemic outcomes.

Keywords

pandemic – affect – affective disorders – security – depression

 | DOI:10.1163/9789004748187_004

1 *In Lieu* of an Introduction: The (Dis)Order of Discourse

> It is the value of all morbid states that they show us under a magnifying glass certain states that are normal – but not easily visible when normal.
>
> F. NIETZSCHE, quoted from G. CANGUILHEM (1991: 45)

> 1.25 million cases. The number of new cases is increasing by over a thousand daily. 9320 fatalities.
>
> World Health Organization, *WHO COVID-19 Dashboard*

These are the painfully surreal numbers for COVID-19 as of the first day of October 2021 – the day this chapter is being written. The numbers that seem to reveal so much and yet so little. What are these numbers really saying? And, more importantly, what are they not saying?

In his lecture "The Order of Discourse," Michel Foucault argues that in order for a proposition to be considered valid, it must be "in the true" (*dans le vrai*)[1] (Foucault 1981: 60). "In the true" is another term for a discursive matrix that establishes the legitimacy of a given proposition within the epistemo-(onto)-logical order of discourse. Foucault notes that "within its own limits, each discipline recognizes true and false propositions." "But it pushes back a whole teratology of knowledge beyond its margins" (Ibid.). Upon reflection of these figures, it is evident that they are valid, truthful, and accurate. However, following Foucault's "repression hypothesis," we must inquire what falls beyond this statistical representation.

In the episteme formed by the natural science paradigm at the end of the nineteenth century, statistics emerged as a principle for verifying propositions' so-called "truthfulness," serving as a tool for validation, simply put, as a "guarantor of the truth." Foucault explains that a new (biological–medical) field of observation emerges "in an infinitely open series of generations, where [the trait, the proposition] appears and disappears according to statistical regularities" (Ibid: 61). Foucault promptly highlights that statistical regularity is a novel means of disciplining discourse, "a principle of control over the production of discourse" (Ibid). The relationship between statistics and discipline is made even more apparent through his lecture series *Security, Territory, Population*, where Foucault describes the mortality rate of smallpox: such that, in the eighteenth century, 1 in every 7,782 people died of this disease (Foucault 2009: 86). A number with very small decimal places indicates a human life – an optimal, precisely calculated, and depersonalized

1 The concept was originally introduced by Foucault's teacher and PhD supervisor George Canguilhem.

number of deaths. The *tertium quid* that unifies statistics and discipline is the norm – the norm provides meaning for the internal rules of (re)producing discourse, otherwise known as *the order of discourse*.

What do the almost 10,000 deaths during the pandemic in Lithuania mean within the discourse? Perhaps the reduction of the *infinitely open* continuum of phenomena to a medical case, a number, a law – and, as a result, a *norm*. Although it could be argued that documenting the pandemic's dynamics, including infections and recoveries, sick and healthy individuals, pre-mortem cases and deaths, in general, positive or negative changes is natural and meaningful, one could answer in Foucault's words that in this case, *the document* turns into a *monument*. The *monumentality of* statistics *qua*, its historical symptomatic significance (Foucault 1972: 137) implies that statistics becomes a metadiscursive tool that trumps the logic of the discourse's "in the true," which, in turn, enables the objectification as a valid discursive practice that eliminates any statement inconsistent with this logic. In simple terms, statistics based on regularity becomes an absolute and unquestioned *norm*.

And yet, what remains beyond the normative order of discourse? In "Mental Health and the COVID-19 Pandemic," Pfefferbaum et al. describe a broad spectrum of affective responses to the COVID-19 pandemic, ranging from the stress caused by the effects of the disease and the fear of infection to more nuanced mental expressions, such as boredom, and agitation, depression, frustration; or even psychosomatic ones, such as insomnia, anxiety, and panic attacks (Pfefferbaum et al.: 2020). The authors exclusively use the negative affective register to describe various *affects* (feelings, emotions, psychosomatic states) experienced by individuals. On one hand, it is possible to identify the mechanism of the same discursive logic, in which "live," singular, and (despite their commonality) individual experiences are transformed into abstract medical terms, symptoms, and diagnostic tools, and become self-explanatory hermetic discursive constructs that *seemingly* require no further elaboration. On the other hand, these accumulative experiences reveal the flaws in the so-called flawless order of discourse. In a sense, they serve as "portals" leading beyond the order established by (and within) discourse, unveiling a new dimension of human existence, challenged by its own limitations. In addition, these experiences encourage us to step away from the medicalized, *ergo* universalized, and normalized approach to understanding the pandemic experience and, instead, to reflect upon the socio-political aspects of such experiences – those that the order of discourse attempts to invisibly exclude from the "true" category of discourse.

Is depression solely a medical symptom, or is it also (and perhaps even more) a social and political symptom? Has the pandemic alone caused such a reaction, or is it also due to its management? Do *articulating* sadness, pain, and fear suffice for their *recognition*? At this stage, these questions might seem premature, especially since the pandemic was an unprecedented event, a kind of socio-political experiment with no prior knowledge of the tools, its course, or results. However, it is precisely the response to the unexpected and the unknown that serves as the best, to put it semi-ironically, a "rapid test" of the actions of political – or, more specifically, biopolitical – power. The *governmentality*[2] – governance – executed by those in power has been impeccably (both politically and economically) rational and prompt, as much as these adjectives are meaningful in such a contingent context. At the outset, the "valid" priorities were identified, security and order, which, as if by a Hegelian synthesis that removes differences and contradictions – are combined into *care*.

At first glance, the trifecta of security, order, and care seems to be a perfectly valid guideline for crisis management in a pandemic. However, biopolitical theories require a more critical examination of the political strategy established by this triad. It must be noted that these three strands of the triad are *universalizing* and, in this sense, nullify the particularity of pandemic experiences despite their efficiency "on paper." Mathew Arthur provides a strikingly apt notion of "sanitizing force" (Arthur 2020: xvii). It is precisely this sanitizing force, which, alongside the material pathogen (the virus), cleanses and removes discursive "foreignness," was used to manage the pandemic. One could argue that the order of discourse hides the *dis*order of the affective (emotional, psychic, and somatic) response to this discourse. The triumph of biopolitical security has translated into existential insecurity for many individuals. Precision-oriented control, disguised as care, became a dangerous form of what Sergei Prozorov calls "unrequited (hence unidirectional and vertical) love" (Prozorov 2007: 54), enabling "caring" control under a "common good" policy. This control includes constant surveillance, regulation, adjustment, optimization, and sometimes even punishment or elimination.

This chapter questions the validity of order, security, and care as foundational principles of pandemic governance, drawing on current theories of biopolitics. Conceptualizing pandemic management and the corresponding discourse as a "sanitizing force" (M. Arthur) will demonstrate: (a) how the pursuit of social security hassled to the denial of *vita activa* (vitality and affirmative nature of life) and the rise of what I conceptualize as "total lockdown" and "sad passions" and (b) how the "encapsulating" discourse has homogenized the

2 Foucault's portmanteau that combines *government/governance* and *mentality*.

broad spectrum of the affective response and reduced it to "total lockdown." The critique of the main aspect of the crisis response to the COVID-19 pandemic is based on Elizabeth Grosz's insight, who argues that "evil is not so much an active power as a deprivation of the good" (Grosz 2017: 81). Thus, deprivation is discussed as a technique of discursive discipline, which involves insensitivity and a lack of recognition of the affective consequences of the pandemic. I argue that this technique displaces intense affective drama behind the "smokescreen" of discursive order.

In the last part of the chapter, I critically reflect on such a discursive configuration and explore alternative extra-/para-/sub-discursive structures. These structures allow for more nuanced infrastructures of feeling (Coleman 2018: 600) and ensure that lived experiences are not reduced to statistical information and medical terminology.

2 Biopolitical Security: Existential (In)Security

> Necropower can take multiple forms: the terror of actual death; or a more "benevolent" form – the result of which is the destruction of a culture in order to "save people" from themselves.
>
> MBEMBE 2003: 22

According to Foucault, security has become a guideline and objective and, thus, a new paradigm of political governance since the nineteenth century, heavily influenced by neoliberal ideology and consolidated in the twentieth century. This shift from the *ancien* to *noveau régime* has clear biopolitical implications. Public health governance, manifested as stringent regulation of epidemic outbreaks during times of crisis, exemplifies the connection between power mechanisms and life. In this scenario, life becomes the target of the power's intervention, surveillance, and control. Under neoliberalism, promoting public health and well-being is not only a political decision but also an economic one. In his lecture series, *Security, Territory, Population*, Foucault utilized a historical–genealogical analysis to demonstrate how the emerging apparatus of security (*dispositif*), which aims to promote the well-being of populations and is thus not only political but also biopolitical, is different from the prior apparatus of discipline because of its conductivity and focus on productivity. The universality of explicit and axiomatic prescriptive schemes, representative of normative discipline (*ancien régime*), is replaced by a processual immanent *normalization*: the technique that involves deriving norms from the environment itself by responding to the overall dynamics and changes in environmental factors. In the next series of lectures titled "The Birth of Biopolitics," Foucault introduces the concept of *laissez-faire* to refer to immanent governmentality, which is the optimal governance approach used in the neoliberal paradigm. This approach is characterized not by over-governing but instead by governing only *as much as required* (Foucault 2004: 130–131).

Foucault connects the alteration of the internal *logic* of governance with a shift in *the object of* governance: in the neoliberal paradigm, which, for him, is synonymous with biopolitics, the target of power is no longer singular individuals but whole populations. In the series *Security, Territory, Population*, the philosopher highlights that people are no longer called humanity (*le genre humaine*) but are instead described as a species of people (*l'espèce humaine*) (Foucault 2009: 105). Needless to say, this labeling has transformed people into a mere biological factor. In contrast to the discipline, which utilized *coercive* mechanisms to subjugate individuals to the power apparatus, biopolitical population management is monitoring-based. To explicate the new monitoring model, Foucault suggests the metaphor of the shepherd and the herd, which Prozorov analyzes in depth. First, Prozorov notes that biopower targets not individual territories but entire populations. Second, he notes the assumption that the herd cannot exist without a shepherd. Third, the question of the legitimacy of authority is rendered meaningless as the shepherd does not need the herd's permission to be supervised. Fourth, Prozorov notes a change in power's logic: while the sovereign was responsible for ruling his people collectively, the shepherd is now responsible for both the flock as a whole and each individual. Finally, the shepherd's power – which involves caring for and sustaining the herd – is presented not as a form of governance but rather as a distinct obligation to cultivate life (Prozorov 2007: 54–55). In the words of Foucault, this mode of governance is *omnes et singulatim* – governing everything and everyone – *par excellence*.

Considering the management of a pandemic, this appears to be the preferred approach since, as the term pandemic (*pan demos*) suggests, it affects *every person directly*. Nevertheless, this *all-encompassing* aspect of a pandemic has also proved to be *universalizing*: the diverse array of existences (as well as life experiences and individual reactions to them) has been compressed into one single description – life – which must be safeguarded (*á la* Foucault's *Society Must Be Defended*). This imperative to maintain (and even defend) life reveals the opposite side of this governmental model: it exposes a distinct vertical power structure as it operationalizes a structuring hierarchical logic. The generic term of apparently good care appears to conceal the crucial reality that the recipients of care (the population and its members) are unable to determine the extent and type of care that is applied to them or refuse it altogether. On the contrary, no alternative types of care have been implemented that would address the adverse affective responses brought on by pandemic management: for instance, fostering a participatory culture (involving citizens in critical political decisions) or providing structured support to individuals who have encountered mental health difficulties or whose mental health problems have been aggravated by the pandemic. Thus, the biopower's care is coercive and conditional, aiming to ensure the welfare of populations only as a means of promoting the biopower's own well-being. Therefore, as Prozorov persuasively asserts, as long as the welfare of the population remains the top priority, we remain inevitably in the territory of negative biopolitics (Prozorov 2007: 66).

Another question that has remained unanswered is: how was the so-called supervision conducted? Lawrence Grossberg's concept of the *affective epidemic* can greatly assist in answering this question. Grossberg applies this concept to everyday life, which, he believes, reflects the power mechanisms at work. He explains that the affective epidemic alters everyday life by redistributing and dispersing a series of affective investments (Grossberg 1992: 294). Affective investments in a particular phenomenon result in shaping the population's feelings, moods, imagination, and hopes – in other words, its affects. The affective epidemic steers otherwise erratic affective flows, shaping the usually free-flowing affective investments. In the words of Gilles Deleuze and Fèlix Guattari, the affective epidemic is a process of territorializing and reterritorializing affects, leading to the formation of what Grossberg calls "affective alliances." According to Martin Bressani, the latter are the *topoi of* the social network that enable individuals to discover themselves and feel a much-needed social sense of belonging (Bressani 2010: 160). Grossberg provides the example of the family (debates about the family, discourse about the family, the family as practice, etc.) as one of the actual sites where affective epidemics occur. To illustrate affective epidemics at work, he cites the campaign against narcotic drugs, carried out by conservatives in the United States with the aim of mobilizing the American people against drugs and creating fear (Grossberg 1992: 284–285).

In political terms, fear, anxiety, stress, despair, and related affective states can be convenient for the power apparatus because they allow it to mobilize populations in a comparatively short period of time and with relatively few resources. Fear is directly correlated with threat, risk, and danger, and an affective epidemic inevitably creates the impression that the fear-inducing phenomenon is everywhere, as was evident in the case of the COVID-19 pandemic. However, the actual scale of the globality of the phenomenon is not the issue (there is no doubt about that). The issue, in terms of discourse theory, is that the discourse is gaining the status of hegemony, so that the unrelenting investment in the affective epidemic is like a smoke screen, obscuring other possible places for affective investment. From this perspective, Grossberg's concept of the affective epidemic and the actual epidemic seem to have an eerie resonance: drawing upon Robert Esposito's conceptual scheme, the biopolitical management of the pandemic itself begins to act as an ideological *contagion*, mimicking the logic of the spread of a virus by "infecting" the members of the population with fear, anxiety, panic, and despair. In a paradoxical manner, this turns the *biopolitical security* of the population into *existential insecurity*.

This paradoxical functioning of biopower is discussed by Patricia Clough and Craig Willes. They term this form of governance as "population racism" that is inextricably linked to the circulation of negative affects. According to Clough and Willes (2010: 49), biopower circulates "insecurity and fear and thereby justifies the exceptional treatment of some populations as a matter of biopolitical manipulation." During a pandemic, insecurity, fear, and other negative affects are not limited to only conventionally vulnerable populations; rather, every individual, each *body* is *a part* of a vulnerable population. By establishing security, which is projected to be comprehensive, the security apparatus exploits the inherent vulnerability of bodies by disguising such a strategy as care, manipulating insecurities, and, to some extent, exploiting and abusing them. Neel Ahuja develops a similar conceptual argument, suggesting that the "vulnerability of humanity to a virtual, alien species (*smallpox virus* – author's remark, D.P.) was deployed to help intensify the public sense of insecurity" (Ahuja 2016: 136).

Another significant aspect of biopolitical pandemic management is highlighted by Brian Massumi, who refers to such a form of governance as "preemption." Preemption involves the management of not only present (actual) phenomena but also possible virtual or potential consequences. When explaining the concept of preemption, Massumi contrasts it with prevention, which tends to be employed when a risk or danger is definitively and objectively existent (Massumi 2015: 5). In contrast, preemption refers to "acting on the time before": before something becomes a clear and present danger" (Massumi 2015: vii). To paraphrase, prevention is grounded in objective knowledge, while preemption involves responding to *uncertainty* and *the unknown* – that is, pure virtuality. The biopolitical intervention takes place in the modality of virtuality characterized by uncertainty and lack of knowledge. Thus, biopower exploits caused by the latter insecurity by offering "protection" in return. This exploitation of insecurity points to what Ericka Tucker calls "affective state disorders" (Tucker 2013: 118).

3 From a State of Lesser to Greater Perfection (and Back)

> This pandemic is the season of "nevertheless."
>
> ADELMAN 2021: 463

Moving away from the biopolitical "contagion," affective epidemics, and ideological viruses, I will further explore a different, more nuanced and sophisticated form of contagion – affect. Such a conceptualization of affect (which, in the most general sense, can be understood as our bodily capacities that enable certain transformations) resonates with the one offered by Agnieszka Wolodzko. According to Wolodzko (2020: 213), the contagiousness of affect is "the onto-episteme-ethical condition of living bodies." What is precisely meant here by "the contagiousness of affect?" One of Baruch Spinoza's (more succinct) understandings of affect is as a modification of the body and ideas. This occurs due to the natural interaction between the body and the world around it and vice versa (Spinoza, vol. 3, *Def. III*). Deleuze expands on Spinoza's understanding of affect and introduces the terms *affectio* and *affectus*. While they both affect the body and ideas, these two categories of affect slightly differ in their effects. Affects–modifications (*affectio*) directly modify or change the body, while the second category of affects (*affectus*) results in either a greater or lesser bodily capacity for action (Deleuze 1988: 49). As the body's capacity to act increases, it moves toward a state of greater perfection. Conversely, a decrease in capacity results in a move toward a state of lesser perfection.

In Prop. XI, Ch. 3, Spinoza refers to the stages of transition described here as pleasure and pain. According to Elizabeth Grosz, neither pain nor pleasure are inherently "good" or "bad"; instead, their value is determined by what these affects *enable us* to do or *prevent us from* doing (Grosz 2017: 80). There is thus no need to "psychologize" affect, as it is not psychological in nature – rather, the emotional expression of affect is the outcome of a particular modification or transition. Moreover, as Deleuze notes, affect belongs to the domain of *ethology* – its effects on the body or *what the body can do* (Deleuze 1988: 26–27).

The question of what the body can do has become one of the most pressing issues in the context of the pandemic. Figuratively speaking, due to "the total lockdown," bodies seem to have lost the trajectory of movement (towards perfection) and to have undergone only negative modifications – sad passions. We found ourselves in a paradoxical situation where we became as distant from each other as possible while, at the same time, being highly dependent on each other, mainly due to the fear of virus transmission. The pandemic and the measures taken for security and "care" have deprived us of our power, productivity, and *joie de vivre* and, in turn, have forced us into a state of existential anxiety, social apathy, and political melancholy. Following Lauren Berlant, this affective configuration could be labeled as "flat affect," in which the vitality and intensity of affect disappear, leaving behind, metaphorically speaking, an "empty shell" (Duschinsky and Wilson 2014: 185). It is important to note, however, that the flatness of affect hides the excessive intensity of the experience that overwhelms and shocks the subject (the body). In an attempt to protect itself from this shock, the body "shuts down" and hides all signs of emotion or feelings. Translated into socio-political terms, the concept of "flat affect" could be referred to as "interpassivity" (Žižek 2006: 23–26), which stands for the indifference that arises from weakness and despair and leads to a lack of initiative to change the situation. This apathy creates mistrust in figures of power and politics in general, ultimately leading to political inertia.

Despite being unable to avoid "sad passions," we should not overlook an equally significant (if not more) dimension that the pandemic has emphasized: the shared experience of *sadness* that was always present in the background. Our shared vulnerability (though varying in intensity among individuals) enables us to adopt an ethical standpoint to affective reactions. As gracefully put by Sara Ahmed, vulnerability exposes our dependence on others, which entails two possible scenarios: either loss and pain or love and protection (Ahmed 2004: 68–69, 125). In other words, we may experience a surge in "sad passions" or a boost in affirmative, empowering affects. And yet, in the face of countless transformations, modifications, and mutations, how can one endure through the unknown while in grief? Rosi Braidotti stresses the importance of perseverance: we must endure the transitions without *cracking* (Braidotti 2012: 175). The core of this ethical principle, which perhaps could even be considered an imperative, is to incorporate cracks and protect oneself (and others) while transitioning between states, not only by enduring each modification but also by attempting to enhance one's own endurance, thus achieving existential affirmation. In summary, one should strive to reestablish a sense of "intimacy with the world" (Braidotti 2016: 51) in a crucial attempt to regain trust in it.

Rebecca Adelman (as if instinctively following Braidotti) refers to the pandemic as the season of *nevertheless* – tensions, contradictions, and ideology (Adelman 2021: 463, 465). Contrary to resilience celebrated by neoliberalism (the capability to recover, regenerate, and restore lost form following deformation or shock), Adelman underscores the significance of endurance. Endurance prevails over resilience because while resilience allows one to withstand adversities, endurance is capable of surviving boredom and monotony, thereby becoming an existential form of "nevertheless" (Adelman 2021: 470). In the words of Donna Haraway, endurance empowers us to "stay with the trouble" (Haraway 2016). Trouble can manifest in various horrifying forms, including the illness or even death of loved ones. However, during pandemics, the trouble mostly took on the form of being cut off from the whole world, claustrophobic confinement to limited space, and exacerbated anxiety, which can ultimately wear down even the most robust and resilient individuals.

The ultimate idea I would like to reflect on in this section is the *inexpressibility* of sadness. Anne Boyer highlights the peculiar aporetic attribute of pain, stating its non-communicative aspect despite being "egalitarian." In other words, pain is inherently non-communicative, and its universality does not diminish (but, on the contrary, enhances) its particularity and singularity (Boyer 2019: 213–214). Nonetheless, pain's "egalitarianism," coupled with our inherent vulnerability and the need for perseverance (*nevertheless*) drives us to not only reconceptualize our relationships with ourselves, with the Other/others, and the pandemic itself but, more importantly, explore new ways, forms, and techniques to understand the pandemic – beyond the confines of the sanitizing discourse. This approach enables us to take *genuine care of* ourselves – something that even the most functional apparatus of security has thus far failed to accomplish (and perhaps never will).

4 *In Lieu* of Conclusions: The (In)Visibility of Depression

> Care is a defiant act.
>
> MATHEW ARTHUR

Raymond Williams, a Marxist literary critic, proposed the concept of structures of feeling, drawing a parallel between the structures of feelings and experiences and the dimension of social relations (Williams 1997: 130). Structures are social, fixed, and mostly universal. Reviewing Williams' concept of structures of feeling, Rebecca Coleman proposed her alternative concept of *infrastructures* of feeling, with two significant additions over the original one. First, infrastructures of feelings focus on the complex architecture and architectonics of feelings, allowing for a conceptual understanding of interconnections, relations, clusters, and the dynamic nature of feelings. Second, infrastructures facilitate the "transmission" of affect into the structure – "how the affectivity of the present is encountered, experienced, and organized" (Coleman 2018: 610–611).

The paradoxical anti-structural aspect of infrastructures of feelings, i.e., *infra-* is what I find most relevant in the pandemic context. Dadaist artist Marcel Duchamp proposes various *affective* conceptualizations of *infra-mechanics*, establishing a barely visible boundary between different objects: ice melting in water, the warmth left behind on a seat, residue of tobacco smoke in one's mouth, the feeling of velvet trousers against one's skin, etc. (Goldsmith 2018). *Infra-* captures small, usually imperceptible, and consciously unrecorded changes that are nonetheless real and bring the present back to its affective, intense, and transformative existential significance. *Infra-* designates the contours of the "lines of flight" – the paths of escape from the claustrophobic order of discourse, which could be both universal and individual.

I would like to provide examples of *a different* experience of the pandemic related to the outlined conceptual infra-vectors. For instance, Matthew Arthur poses a valid question: how should we (re)write a pandemic? (Arthur 2020: vi). Arthur suggests an auto/ethnographic approach to living in a pandemic, allowing us to cope with the pandemic's claustrophobic experience, both physically (living in a confined space) and discursively. Such an approach *queers* the sense of space and time (Arthur 2020: xviii), intensifying (revitalizing) the homogenized everyday life. Arthur suggests a repertoire of various para-discursive devices to discover the hidden micro-events in the tedious daily routine of the pandemic, creating infrastructures of multiple relations that connect people with themselves and others while overcoming limiting factors. For example, mask-making, metaphorically speaking, functions like infra-power, connecting people across physical distance by 'exporting' care and encouraging us to explore unconventional forms of community that challenge even spatial constraints. Furthermore, as noted by Arthur, such practices may disrupt the supposedly flawless social "hygiene," transforming carefully curated social relations into a tangled web of trust (Arthur 2020: viii).

In a world that has lost, in Arthur's words, its "materiality," such micro-practices reconfigure our typical ways of experiencing and relating to the world, not in quantitative terms (as both the pandemic itself and its management have already done), but in qualitative terms. For instance, reading groups on *Skype* establish nuanced synchronic infrastructures that connect bodies, institutions, media, and technologies in a diachronic passing of time. The cultivation of plants for domestic use challenges capitalist modes of production. The creation of neologisms to describe the pandemic (such as *blursday* and *quaranteams*) provides a new conceptual language as an alternative to the pandemic's hegemonic discourse.

Linda Barry's graphic project *Documenting All the Small Things That Are Easily Lost* (2020) also emphasizes the significance of the everyday. The artist produces a visual self-therapeutic diary, best described by the rhetorical question, "how did then become now"? At the heart of this graphic diary lies the dialectic of discovery and loss, which, during the pandemic, presented itself as the disruption of normal, comfortable life and the consequent realization of one's self in an unfamiliar, claustrophobic (both limiting and empowering) assemblage. To combat claustrophobia, forced isolation, and the monotony of quarantine, she documents significant moments, reflects on her existence, and describes her experiences, thoughts, and fears in detail. She also uses affirmations, reminders, and selective yet meaningful silences as a means of resistance. This project highlights the ability to act, live, and appreciate life "nevertheless," underscoring the resistance that emerges through everyday life and the anti-moralistic dynamic between past, present, and future selves. Ultimately, it suggests that *it's okay to feel bad.*

The expression "it's okay to feel bad," now a pandemic "mantra," enables us to transition from individual pandemic experiences to a more universal understanding. How can we define collective sadness and emerge from it in solidarity in times of grief? Anna Cvetkovich, a philosopher, created *The Alphabet of Feeling Bad*, a complex artistic initiative, first displayed in 2012 but revisited during the pandemic. The project presents each letter of the alphabet corresponding to negative emotion and captures them in material artifacts, such as a messy bed, billboards, and political clothing bearing political slogans promoting a "brighter tomorrow," ethnographic displays, books on critical gender and race theory, and various other artistic works. Feelings, such as guilt, shame, isolation, and fear of being misunderstood, associated with feeling bad, typically concealed individually or publicly invisible, form the range of emotions in *The Alphabet of Feeling Bad* exhibition. The philosopher explores alternative forms of unity and community by employing artistic techniques to establish a backdrop. This, together with the use of critical autoethnography and narratology, provides a glimpse into the union based on collective negative experiences yet considering individuality, singularity, and personhood.

The umbrella term for this ethnographic project is depression, which Cvetkovich refers to as a "public feeling" in her book. Cvetkovich's observation that depression is not only a medical issue but also a socio-political one is apt: depression is not only a medical or biochemical dysfunction of the individual (in this case, the burden of it falls entirely on the sufferer) but rather a symptom of the surrounding environment (Cvetkovich 2012: 25–26). Adopting this approach frees us from the hold of pathologizing discourse and encourages critical reflection on the discursive tools used to distinguish "normal" and "abnormal" behavior. It also empowers us to reject accusations that function as interpellations and reclaim what Cvetkovich calls "sovereignty of feeling," as she emphasized in one of her lectures, which she delivered during a global pandemic. The sovereignty of feeling, in the case of depression, has not only individual emancipatory potential but also significant collective implications. Depression, as noted by Cvetkovich, may manifest as typically considered anti-social behavior like withdrawal or inertia. However, it can also lead to the emergence of new and alternative social dynamics that enable different types of relationships, connections, and patterns of collectivity (Cvetkovich 2012: 6).

The pandemic exposed common vulnerabilities, insecurities, and existential fragility among people and stirred sad passions. The collective response to it was a shaky balance between care and protest. Emerging as a form of inner protest, a productive form of *care* as a *protest* emerged, directed mainly against the discourse that objectifies everything. Perhaps this experience could remind us about another potential scenario: *protest* taking the shape of *care*.

References

Adelman, R. 2021. "Enduring COVID-19, nevertheless," *Cultural Studies* 25 (2–3): 462–474.

Ahmed, S. 2004. *The Cultural Politics of Emotions*. Edinburgh: Edinburgh University Press.

Ahuja, N. 2016. *Bioinsecurities: Disease Interventions, Empire, and the Government of Species*. Durham and London: Duke University Press.

Arthur, M. 2020. "Care is a Defiant Act: Writing Pandemic Feels," *Capacious: Journal for Emerging Affect Inquiry* 2 (1–2): vi–xviii.

Boyer, A. 2019. *The Undying: Pain, Vulnerability, Mortality, Medicine, Art, Time, Dreams, Data, Exhaustion, Cancer, and Care*. New York: Farrar, Straus and Giroux.

Braidotti, R. 2012. "Nomadic Ethics." In Smith, Daniel, Somers-Hall Henry (eds.). *The Cambridge Companion to Deleuze*. Cambridge: Cambridge University Press, 170–197.

Braidotti, R. 2016. "Posthuman Affirmative Politics." In. *Resisting Biopolitics: Philosophical, Political, and Performative Strategies*. New York: Routledge, 30–56.

Bressani, M. 2010. "Towards a Digital Theory of Affect," *ACADIA. Life in: formation*, 159–163. Available via the Internet: http://papers.cumincad.org/data/works/att/acadia10_159.content.pdf [accessed 2022-10-15].

Canguilhem, G. 1991. *The Normal and the Pathological*, translated by Carolyn Fawcett. New York: Zone Books.

Clough, P.; Willse, C. 2010. "Gendered Security / National Security: Political Branding and Population Racism," *Social Text* 28 (4): 49.

Coleman, R. 2018. "Theorizing the present: digital media, pre-emergence and infrastructures of feeling," *Cultural Studies* 32 (4): 600–622.

Cvetkovich, A. 2012. *Depression as a Public Feeling*. London and Durham: Duke University Press.

Deleuze, G. 1988. *Spinoza: Practical Philosophy*, translated by R. Hurley. San Francisco: City Lights Books.

Duschinsky, R.; Wilson, E. 2014. "Flat Affect, Joyful Politics, and Enthralled Attachments: Engaging with the Work of Lauren Berlant," *International Journal of Politics, Culture, and Society* 28 (3): 179–190.

Esposito, R. 2011. *Immunitas: The Protection and Negation of Life*, translated by Z. Hanafi. Cambridge: Polity Press.

Foucault, M. 1972. *The Archeology of Knowledge and the Discourse on Language*, translated by A. M. Sheridan Smith. New York: Pantheon Books.

Foucault, M. 1986. "Omnes et Singulatim: Towards a Critique of Political Reason," *Le Dèbat* 41 (4): 5–36.

Foucault, M. 1981. "the Order of Discourse." In Young, Robert (ed.). *Untying the text: a Post-Structuralist Reader*. London: Routledge, 48–78.

Foucault, M. 2003. *Society Must Be Defended: Lectures at the College de France 1975–1976*, translated by. D. Macey. New York: Picador.

Foucault, M. 2004. *The Birth of Biopolitics, Lectures at the College de France 1978–1979*, translated by G. Burchell. New York: Palgrave Macmillan.

Foucault, M. 2009. *Security, Territory, Population: Lectures at the College de France 1977–1978*, translated by G. Burchell. New York: Palgrave Macmillan.

Goldsmith, K. 2018. *1000 infrathins*. Pennsylvania: The Center for Programs in Contemporary Writing.

Grossberg, L. 1992. *We Gotta Get out of This Place: Popular Conservatism and Postmodern Culture*. New York and London: Routledge.

Grosz, E. 2017. *The Incorporeal: Ontology, Ethics, and the Limits of Materialism*. New York: Columbia University Press.

Haraway, D. 2016. *Staying with the Trouble: Making Kin in the Chthulucene*. Durham: Duke University Press Books.

Massumi, B. 2015. *Ontopower: War, Powers, and the State of Perception*. Durham, London: Duke University Press.

Mbembe, A. 2003. "Necropolitics", translated by L. Meintjes, *Public Culture* 15 (1): 11–40.

Pfeffebraum, B., et al. 2020. "Mental Health and the Covid-19 Pandemic", *The New England Journal of Medicine* 383 (6): 510–512.

Prozorov, S. 2007. "The Unrequited Love of Power: Biopolitical Investment and the Refusal of Care," *Foucault Studies* 4: 53–77.

Spinoza, B. 2001. *The Ethics*, translated by R. H. M. Elwes. Blackmask Online.

Tucker, E. 2013. "Affective Disorders of the State: A Spinozian Diagnosis and Cure," *Journal of East-West Thought* 3 (3): 97–119.

Williams, R. 1977. *Marxism and Literature*. Oxford: Oxford University Press.
Wolodzko, A. 2020. "Living within affect as contamination: breathing in between numbers," *Capacious: Journal for Emerging Affect Inquiry* 2 (1–2): 212–224.
Žižek, S. 2006. *How to Read Lacan*. London: Granta Books.

CHAPTER 3

Pandemic and Race: Un(fore)seen Circumstances, Same Old Biopolitics?

Aistis Žekevičius

Abstract

This chapter suggests that, instead of opening unexpected paths towards a better understanding of mutual interconnectedness and vulnerability, pandemic biopolitics exacerbates the existing structural racial inequality by reinforcing the necropolitical regimes of exclusion and amplifying the workings of racialization in biopolitics. First, the chapter analyzes the biopolitical uses of race before moving on to discern the general capitalization of life and highlight the colonial nature of epidemiology. Second, it focuses on the neoliberal subjectivity of the new working class and argues that the Foucauldian imperative "make live or let die" gave way to the differentiation between lives to be saved and lives to be risked in pandemic biopolitics. Third, the chapter claims that the COVID-19 pandemic has exposed the race-based necropolitics of usable bodies and the biopolitics based on the distribution of differential vulnerability. Finally, it turns to decolonial, politico-economic, ecological, and solidary remedies that might help us find solutions to the current necropolitical impasse.

Keywords

biopolitics – necropolitics – pandemic – race – vulnerability

1 Introduction

Even if one were to relegate the political sphere entirely and go by the biological in the face of the global COVID-19 pandemic, the evidence that testifies to the link between the pandemic and race is striking. Several studies suggest that the mortality burden of the pandemic hit racial and/or ethnic minorities the most, thus underscoring the importance of the social determinants of health in the face of a public health crisis (Aburto et al. 2022, Silverio et al. 2022, Solomos 2021). A medical study by Justin M. Feldman and Mary T. Bas-

 | DOI:10.1163/9789004748187_005

sett focused entirely on the effects of race, ethnicity, and education on mortality due to COVID-19 and its complications found that mortality rates among most racial and ethnic minorities in the United States were much higher than the mortality of non-Hispanic whites within the same age group. Furthermore, were all racial and ethnic groups to have the same conditions as the latter, the mortality rate from COVID-19 and its complications within racial and ethnic minorities would have been 71% lower (Feldman and Bassett 2021). This encourages one to take a closer look at what lies behind these statistics, which may otherwise be explained by referring to supposedly innate racial differences, and tackle the issues related to the pandemic and race not in the biological but rather in the politico-philosophical sense. And it is precisely here that the category of biopolitics makes its unexpected return to the forefront of philosophical debates, as the claim that the pandemic has ultimately illuminated and intensified racial inequalities around the world is supported by a number of theorists (Butler 2022: 4, 65; Boukalas 2023: 97; Randolph 2021: 8; Ristić, Marinković 2022: 3; Solomos 2021: 725–726).

While some philosophers accurately point out the theoretical and political shortcomings of biopolitics either as a general instrument of critique (Breu 2013: 49) or, more specifically, as a tool to address the COVID-19 pandemic (Lorenzini 2020: S40), many theorists agree that biopolitics made its return as an important analytical tool precisely because of the fact that many world countries have decided to enforce strict political measures in order to prevent the spread of the global pandemic. In a series of essays written around the outbreak of the pandemic, Giorgio Agamben was quick to react in a somewhat explosive manner by claiming that the epidemic was "invented" by the biopower to extend its grasp and expand the state of exception beyond any limitations (Agamben 2021: 12). Others, for instance, Jean-Luc Nancy, argued for a more lenient approach to the measures enforced by states, suggesting that the pandemic is a biological, computer-scientific, and cultural exception, which requires equally exceptional measures (Nancy 2021: 27). But the relationship between the pandemic and biopolitics is perhaps most concisely defined by Jesús Ayala-Colqui, who claims: "It would be a mistake to reduce this early 21st-century pandemic to a mere biological fact, to a clinical dilemma, to a natural question, for it is also a political phenomenon, in the strictest sense. The COVID-19 pandemic is political insofar as it requires extraordinary government intervention in order to manage it, and also because those actionsmust be inserted into an existing mechanism of governmentality that affects human, non-human and natural biological life" (Ayala-Colqui 2020: 379). And while some thinkers prefer to analyze the pandemic by invoking other notions[1] – Christos Boukalas, for instance, locates the shift from the biopolitical management of life to the management of threat and thereby prefers to speak of threat governmentality as a new modality of power, which is founded on the ontological certainty of the threat – it is clear that biopolitics, once thought to have retreated from the epicenter of philosophy, must be revisited once again (Boukalas 2023: 142–146, emphasis in original).

To reconsider the troubled relationship between the pandemic and race, several related notions and ideas are revisited in this text. First, the issues of biopolitical use(s) of race, the capitalization of life, and the coloniality of public health are being addressed by analysing the ideas of feminist, queer and race scholar Sara Ahmed, economist Gary Becker, and epidemiologist Eugene T. Richardson. Then, my focus turns to the questions regarding the neoliberal subjectivity of the new working class in pandemic conditions, situational vulnerability, and ecology as I take a closer look at works by economic geographer David Harvey, philosopher and gender theorist Judith Butler, and Slovenian cultural theorist Slavoj Žižek. Later, the attention turns to the ideas of Kandida Purnell and her proposed notion of necropolitics of usable bodies, as well as Daniele Lorenzini's biopolitics of differential vulnerability. Finally, the question of possible remedies – decolonial, politico-economic, ecological, and solidary ways to resist necropolitical tendencies of the contemporary governmentality and the structural racial inequality, and challenge the biopolitical status quo itself – is raised, with the help of ideas proposed by Richardson, Harvey, Butler, Cameroonian philosopher Achille Mbembe, and political philosopher Myisha Cherry.

2 On the Biopolitical Use(s) of Race, the Capitalization of Life, and the Coloniality of Epidemiology

Oftentimes, even the most complex analyses can be reduced to one or two simple questions. In this case, the question could be formulated as follows: What is the use of race in pandemic biopolitics? I borrow the concept of use from Ahmed, who analyses how use became associated with life and strength in nineteenth-century biological and social thought in her book *What's the Use? On the Uses of Use*, allowing one to read some of its fragments from the biopolitical viewpoint. Ahmed describes use as a contact zone and introduces

1 Others, for instance, Btihaj Ajana, distinguish between the politics of defense and the politics of sacrifice (Ajana 2021).

the notion of use in the field of biopolitics by claiming that "a question of whose life matters is bound up with who gets to use what" (Ahmed 2019: 40). She argues that one cannot live one's life in isolation, that is, without coming into close contact with things. In the case of COVID-19, however, living one's life without coming into direct contact with another quickly became a privilege, often distributed along the lines of the existing structural inequality. In the pandemic context, race might be seen as a vehicle for categorization, which is introduced by creating "a set of expectations of who will be useful for what, of what some bodies are for or how some bodies become for, of who and what becomes available as resources to be used up" (Ahmed 2019: 95, 136–138, emphasis in original). Here, race is seen as a lens that helps define which bodies are useful and which are set to become disposable, since their utility, conceived of as a system for extracting life even from the death of those deemed a lower class, can be extricated through death by rendering both lives and deaths as resources. Thus, the central biopolitical question regarding the process of making live and letting die becomes tied to social expectations concerning the notions of use and usefulness.

Neoliberal biopolitical regimes, known for their potential to extract life not only from the "wretched of the earth," as Franz Fanon would have it, but virtually from all populations despite their race or class, allow for bringing the category of use into the vocabulary of economics. American economist Gary Becker introduces the concept of the statistical value of life, in which he defines as "the willingness to pay for improvements in probabilities of surviving to different ages," thereby highlighting the connection between the likelihood of staying alive as long as possible and economic power (Becker 2007: 407). And while willingness and probabilities matter, the ability to pay depends on the actual resources available. The definition of the value of life in terms of willingness to pay for it not only allows for transferring most of the responsibility for one's health to the individual but also acknowledges, albeit indirectly, that not all lives are equally valuable and therefore important. In the context of COVID-19, one quote from Becker is particularly telling. More than a decade ago, when considering the possibility of a global avian flu pandemic, he argued that: "While this is an enormous loss, how much precautionary actions are justified depends on the probability of having such a serious pandemic. If the probability of having a pandemic of the same order of severity as the flu pandemic of 1918–19 during the next decade is 1/1000, then the expected worldwide loss in the value of lives would be about $100 billion, which is big enough to justify hurry up efforts to develop vaccines and other protections. On the other hand, if the probability of such a pandemic is only 1/100,000, then the expected worldwide loss is only

$1 billion, and crash vaccine and other programs do not seem urgent" (Becker 2007: 404). What is perhaps the most shocking here is not Becker's explanation of the lack of readiness for such a global pandemic itself, but rather the overall tendency to make far-reaching healthcare decisions, which in the event of a pandemic become crucial in solving the fundamental dilemma of biopolitics – either to boost the chances of surviving or leave one to die – by following the logic of capital, allowing one to speak of a rise of the general capitalization of both public health and life itself. American post-structuralist Judith Butler calls a tendency to apply such logic "a post-sovereign or neo-sovereign form of calculation". According to her, such calculation brings about "a form of inequality that itself relies upon a metric of grievability – whose life, if lost, would count as a loss, enter into the registers of loss, even broach the status of an incalculable loss. And whose death can be quietly calculated without ever being named as such" (Butler 2022: 85–86). Ultimately, the post- or neo-sovereign calculation depends first and foremost on an unequal distribution of grief, which allows her to coin the neologism *differential grievability*. If anything, these quiet deaths only prove that social inequality, which is all too often inseparable from structural racial inequality, goes hand in hand with necropolitical violence.

Of course, one may object to treating health as human capital by claiming that despite the prevalence of economic inequality, there still are certain public healthcare mechanisms that aim to prevent pandemics. However, many of these healthcare programs merit stern postcolonial criticism. American epidemiologist Eugene T. Richardson treats public health first and foremost as an apparatus of colonialism, which perpetuates and exploits global health inequalities through empirical models of infectious disease causation that mostly serve the protected and the wealthy, thereby only further entrenching racial and social inequality in the contemporary matrix of power (Richardson 2020: 4). For Richardson, colonialism is a certain kind of conceptual apparatus that is first and foremost perceived as a matrix of power relations, which manifests itself continuously, transnationally, and intersubjectively by ignoring the statehood of former colonies, and includes not only class, political, economic, or social, but also racial orders imposed by European colonialism, which, having survived decolonization, continue to serve the needs of global capital accumulation to this day (Richardson 2020: 3–4). Yet perhaps the most robust part of his critique is aimed at what Richardson calls the epidemic of illusions – an epidemic that is being spread by the colonialism of knowledge production, supported by certain mechanisms of public health science, especially epidemiology, and particularly its tendency to monopolize the discourse of truth. By linking the concept of coloniality to theories of symbolic coercion and the problem of truth-telling, Richardson highlights the importance of separating epidemiological knowledge production from the neocolonial power matrix (Richardson 2020: 5, 65–88). The imperial and colonial roots of modern epidemic disease control are further highlighted in the latest study by American sociologist and historian of medicine and race Alexandre White, *Epidemic Orientalism: Race, Capital, and the Governance of Infectious Disease*. Referring to the complex of global responses to epidemic threats in terms of supranational dynamics of political, economic, and health relations, White introduces the concept of *epidemic orientalism* to account for the limitations in thought and action that this dominant discursive frame in infectious disease control imposes. Modifying Edward Said's notion of orientalism, White criticizes the predominance of European and Western exceptionalism, colonialism, and racial capitalism in modern infectious disease control, on one hand, and the tendency to reposition the colonial world as a locus of infectious disease threat, on the other hand, which ultimately leads to the classification and categorization of difference that helps to reify the distinctions between the modern West and the rest, reproduce systems of racial difference and colonial exploitation, and establish a teleological model of evaluation and comparison (2023: 17–29). While it is true that not every biomedical intervention into the lives of populations living in colonial spaces is harmful as such, the exceptional nature of these interventions, marked by the racial difference, places White epistemically closer to the likes of Mbembe, Spivak, Chakrabarty, and other critics of modernity than conventional biopolitical theorists, such as Foucault or Agamben.

And while it is true that instead of functioning as an ideological apparatus that represents dominant interests, epidemiology had better parameterize the effects of slavery, exploitative colonialism, targeted underdevelopment, structural regulation, resources extraction, illicit financial flows, and gender-based violence, the postcolonial critique of public health should by no means be limited to the sphere of knowledge production. The COVID-19 pandemic has revealed that some deaths are way quieter than others, and race becomes the crucial factor in this equation more often than not.

3 Neoliberal Subjectivity, Situational Vulnerability, and Ecological Conundrums

Most personal experiences of the pandemic are hardly separable from the state of being ill. In *Spaces of Hope*, a study of globalization and the working body in late twentieth-century capitalism, British economic geographer David

Harvey has observed that illness is primarily defined as an inability to work in capitalism (Harvey 2000: 106). However, when the COVID-19 pandemic broke out, it became apparent that representatives of the so-called "essential jobs" are unable to work remotely and, due to their precarious position, cannot allow themselves not to work, even as it became increasingly dangerous to their own chances of surviving at the height of the pandemic. In one of his more recent articles, Harvey claims that the workforce that is expected to care for the growing number of patients, or at least provide the minimum services to restore daily life throughout the pandemic, is typically heavily gendered, racialized, and ethnicized. Labeling these people as "the new working class," Harvey notes that the representatives of this new working class are facing a double threat: they are constantly accompanied by the greatest risk of contracting the virus while working, on one hand, and the possibility of being fired due to the economic austerity imposed by the pandemic, on the other hand (2020). Such a double threat results in a paradox that contains an ugly choice: they either risk getting infected while caring for others and maintaining basic supplies, or end up being unemployed and potentially losing access to adequate health care, thus bearing the brunt of a situation, in which, as UK-based political philosopher Christos Boukalas has aptly noticed, "biosecurity sacrifices the life *in* the factory in order to secure the life *of* the factory" (Boukalas 2023: 141, emphasis in original). To do so, certain bodies must be designated as acceptable losses despite living productive lives. As members of this workforce have long been socialized to behave as humble and obedient neoliberal subjects, they tend to blame themselves or God when faced with setbacks, and never dare to think that the causes of the problem may lie within the system itself (Harvey 2020). And yet, even they manage to notice they are carrying a disproportionately large burden while maintaining the reproduction of the social order. This brings back into focus the differentiation between lives to be saved and lives to be risked, which embodies the distinction between the political and the physical dimensions of life, as suggested by French anthropologist Didier Fassin as early as 2007 (Fassin 2007: 501). However, these two dimensions can no longer be distinguished in the complex interplay between pandemic and race, as the political and the physical, or the corporeal, dimensions of life become intertwined due to un(fore)seen circumstances of the pandemic.

Naturally, the need to choose between "the life in the factory and the life of the factory" means that any efforts to counter racial inequality tend to be hampered in pandemic times. In her newest book, *What World Is This?*, Butler analyses how COVID-19 and all its political, social, ecological, and economic consequences have challenged us to reconsider the sense of the world that such calamities bring about. Butler locates the issue of the so-called "essential jobs" at the very heart of the "health of the economy vs. health of the population" debate, which arose at the breakout of the pandemic, thereby suggesting that those who advocate for the primacy of the economy in the face of a deadly virus accept the idea that human life must be sacrificed for the economic well-being. Moreover, Butler notices that those modes of reasoning that maintain the need to keep industry and workplaces intact give a new form to the fundamental contradiction inherent to the relationship between wage labor and the worker's immiseration, which Karl Marx has explicated in his *Economic and Philosophic Manuscripts of 1844*: "We open the economy – or keep it open – in order to sustain the lives of the working poor, but the working poor are those whose lives are deemed dispensable by opening the economy, whose work can be replaced by other workers, whose lives do not count as singular and invaluable [...] In other words, under the pandemic conditions, the worker goes to work in order to live, but work is precisely what hastens the worker's death" (Butler 2022: 49–50). But what does that mean from the standpoint of the broader biopolitical perspective? Apparently, the classic Foucauldian "making live and letting die" formula seems not to be working anymore, at least not under pandemic conditions, as those populations who were disproportionately exposed to illness and death were precisely those who were not only left without adequate healthcare but also had no choice except continuing their work; in order to keep on living, they were forced to face death every day, often without adequate means of protection from the deadly virus. Perhaps these dynamics can be best summarized by applying the concept of *situational vulnerability*. First introduced by Australian philosopher Catriona Mackenzie, who has distinguished a distinctive taxonomy of different sources (inherent, situational, and pathogenic) and states (dispositional and occurrent) of vulnerability, situational vulnerability acknowledges the ontological vulnerability that is inherent in the human condition and thereby allows one to identify context-specific forms of vulnerability (Mackenzie 2014: 7). The concept of situational vulnerability is further developed by Austrian social and political philosopher Gottfried Schweiger, who claims that due to the situational vulnerability, some groups of people who are unjustly left unprotected are far more likely to contract the virus, or not get sufficient treatment if they get sick due to social factors that may amount to pathogenic vulnerability (Schweiger 2022: 3). In the context of the COVID-19 pandemic, it seems to be precisely the case with structural racial inequality, as the existing imbalances are further exacerbated in pandemic times.

Last but not least, the interplay between pandemic and race is also inseparable from ecological issues, at least to some extent. In a series of books dedicated to the outbreak of COVID-19 and consisting of short essays, Slovenian philosopher Slavoj Žižek treats the pandemic in a slightly Vonnegutian manner by seeing it as a cynical reminder of "the ultimate contingency and meaninglessness of our lives: no matter how magnificent the spiritual edifices we, humanity, construct, a stupid natural contingency like a virus or an asteroid can end it all [...] not to mention the lesson of ecology, which is that we, humanity, can also unknowingly contribute to this end" (Žižek 2020a: 52). He argues that today's fundamental ideological and political struggle is first and foremost related to the interrelationship of the pandemic, the ecological crisis, and racism. While it is true that the global privileged try to keep these three areas separate from each other and sometimes even hint at the underlying tensions between them, one should persistently maintain the idea of the unity of these three areas, since the spread of epidemics, broadly speaking, is not merely a health problem but is also related to an unbalanced relationship with the natural environment. Žižek agrees that some lives are more meaningless than others, as the representatives of the black race are more vulnerable than most whites, who were able to afford self-isolation and better healthcare during the peak of the pandemic. However, if one were to accept the inherent meaninglessness of human life, this would undermine the very *use* of the ideological and political struggle as proposed by Žižek – and the entire universal healthcare system, in fact. Finally, Žižek argues that the three interrelated crises – epidemiological, ecological, and racial – are produced by the driving forces of global capitalism and were not only predicted by the leading scholars but have been with us for decades (Žižek 2020b: 71–72). Ultimately, it allows one to raise reasonable doubts about the "newness" of the entire plight of the pandemic in terms of both the neoliberal subjectivity of the new working class and the global ecological crisis itself.

4 The Necropolitics of Usable Bodies and the Biopolitics of Differential Vulnerability in the Pandemic

However, with all due respect, the shift towards capitalization of life and the rise of situational vulnerability, which became evident in the wake of the COVID-19 pandemic, seems anything but natural. In her newest study, *Rethinking the Body in Global Politics: Bodies, Body Politics, and the Body Politic in a Time of Pandemic*, London-based political sociologist Kandida Purnell turns to the visual-emotional politics embodied through the COVID-19 pandemic and the fleshing out of contemporary necro(body)politics in order to analyse the relationship between the body and global politics. Drawing on the concept of slow death, formulated by American cultural theorist Lauren Berlant, which describes the physical exhaustion of a given population and the deterioration of its health as a near-defining condition of both its experience and historical existence, Purnell claims that the COVID-19 pandemic has accelerated socio-politically conditioned but usually slower deaths by revealing the extent of the current race, class and gender inequality, thus acting as a mere catalyst of structural inequality (Berlant 2007: 754; Purnell 2021: 79, 129, 138). For Purnell, race is one of the key mechanisms of today's necropolitical logic that brings us back to the notion of use by categorizing bodies according to their usable parts, which thereby can be used until death. According to this logic, it is precisely the fact that there is far less basis for formal complaining about the bodies at the bottom of the global endoskeleton that is responsible for the availability of these bodies to be used and abused by global capital – and discarded as waste without any sense of responsibility and feelings of guilt (Purnell 2021: 80–81). By consuming and disposing of bodies under the guise of "essential services" and placing these people in a confrontation with the power of death to profit others, the necropolitical logic, with the help of overlapping racialized, gendered, and classed classification technologies, disembodies people and transforms them into mere functional parts that serve other bodies during the pandemic. Due to the extractive and exploitative nature of such exchanges, in which other bodies are sought to be freed and preserved, these parts are gradually used and consumed. And because of the insatiable desire to calculate, value, extract, use, and dispose of every animate and inanimate thing, a desire that is peculiar to the modern neoliberal capitalist necropolitics, all populations are ultimately depleted and reduced to numbers and statistics (Purnell 2021: 83–85). While Purnell paints a rather bleak picture of the pandemic, the statistics that illustrate the impact of race, ethnicity, and education on mortality from COVID-19, provided at the introduction of the chapter, seem strongly supportive of these statements.

To characterize such a status quo, distinguished by conditions of slow death and necropolitical outcomes of pandemic biopolitics, Norwegian researcher Tony Sandset has coined the term "state of acceptance" (Sandset 2021: 1411–1412). Modifying the biopolitical notion of the state of exception, first popularized by Agamben and later used by Esposito, Mbembe, and other theoreticians of biopolitics, Sandset claims that the necropolitics of global health inequality is largely driven by a state of chronic acceptance that some simply have poorer health than others. By creating zones where people are exposed to conditions conducive to slow death, pandemic biopolitics keep producing and reproducing necropolitical conditions. Yet another layer to the analysis of the pandemic from the necropolitical standpoint is added by US-based philosopher Daniele Lorenzini, who introduces the concept of differential vulnerability to the discussion of the workings of race in pandemic biopolitics. Building on Michel Foucault's conception of racism as "primarily a way of introducing a break into the domain of life that is under power's control: the break between what must live and what must die" (Foucault 2003: 254), he emphasizes the importance of the differential exposure of human beings to health and social risks, which, for Foucault, is the principal feature of biopolitical governmentality. By contesting a clear-cut biopolitical opposition of life and death, Lorenzini suggests rethinking biopolitics as an effort to differentiate the entire gray spectrum between life and death. For Lorenzini, "biopolitics is always a politics of *differential vulnerability*," a politics that not only is not interested in reducing the existing social and racial inequalities but also "structurally relies on the establishment of hierarchies in the value of lives, producing and multiplying vulnerability as a means of governing people" (Lorenzini 2020: S42–S44, emphasis in original). However, it should be clarified that Lorenzini sees biopolitics first and foremost as a form of injustice, "an *unjust* system of differential vulnerabilities," and is calling for a critical theory of biopolitical rights whose normativity would be seen as rooted in biopolitical technologies of power (Lorenzini 2024: 29, emphasis in original). Using this newly formed theory as a helpful diagnostic and critical tool, specific forms of injustice in our society could be avoided, and our own biopolitical rights could be implemented in a more systematic way, instead of remaining in the vicious circle of the necropolitical production of structural social and racial inequality. And while Lorenzini's suggestions offer much-needed hope, it is concrete solutions one is seeking the most in times of crisis.

5 Looking for Remedies: Decolonial, Politico-economic, Ecological, and Solidary Strategies

Each crisis asks for a working solution, just as each illness demands a search for a cure. There are seemingly at least four types of possible remedies for the current maladies, inseparable from the workings of what one could refer to as the biopolitics of extraction and use: decolonial, politico-economic, ecological, and solidary. Today, when it is no longer possible to reduce complex biopolitical phenomena to one particular cause, and those who choose – whether consciously or not – to remain within the confines of the classic juxtaposition between the health of the population and the autonomy of the individual risk slipping into the realm of conspiracy theories, one must admit that these perspectives, which may appear rather diverse at first sight, are often interrelated, taking over certain elements from each other.

The first – decolonial – cure is offered by Richardson, who notes that the relentless spread of the COVID-19 virus has brought the interconnectedness of humanity into the forefront, hoping that the awareness of this fact will help fight institutionalized racism and ensure truly universal healthcare. Richardson argues that pandemicity, which he conceives of as the binding of humanity through contagion, will potentially make the descendants of colonists aware of the interconnectedness of the world's populations, just as the disproportionate mortality from COVID-19 is the daily experience of much of the global South, where almost 10,000 children die every single day due to entirely avoidable reasons. Perhaps the global North, struck by the newly acquired awareness, would then begin to understand its actual contribution to the production and reproduction of structural injustice and racial inequality and realize that a response to every local outbreak of communicable disease should be as prompt as it was in the case of COVID-19, as the pandemic has illustrated that every local epidemic can easily become a problem of the entire humanity (Richardson 2020: 139–144). However, Richardson himself remains quite sceptical about this possibility and does not rule out the likelihood that militaristic, xenophobic, and necropolitical tendencies may keep gathering momentum in today's world – and I must agree that the possibility of such enlightenment among the ruling elites of the global North sounds rather optimistic and is not entirely reasonable.

The second – politico-economic – solution is suggested by Harvey, who offers what could be labeled as a good old-fashioned socialist prescription while considering ways to change the status quo. He sees the pandemic as an opportunity to unleash the imagination, break free from the oppression of alienating labor, and create a new social order that would take over capitalism's science, technology, and productivity (Harvey 2020). While Harvey's ideas sound truly optimistic in the increasingly necropolitical pandemic landscape, it does not seem that the apparent collapse of capitalism has managed to become even a remote possibility since his predictions about a "collapsing bourgeois society" appeared in 2020. On the contrary, judging from the experience of the COVID-19 pandemic, it seems that after its latest crisis in 2008, capitalism has learned its main lessons and become much more flexible and efficient – and thus able to survive global crises and deal with them in a more productive way that is less harmful to its own workings.

The third – ecological – strategy is proposed by Mbembe, who perceives the pandemic as a spectacular expression of the planetary impasse in which humanity finds itself today. He stresses the inherent oneness of humanity as such and biosphere, considers the restoration of a habitable Earth as the only solution to environmental problems, and proposes the idea that all human beings, regardless of all racial, sexual, civil, and religious differences, are not only the representatives of a single species but are also inseparable from other forms of life (Mbembe 2021c: S62). Quite unexpectedly, Mbembe presents a humanist version of the Stieglerian program, consisting of several strategies that could be adopted to maximize universal equality and prosperity. The first of these is concerned with the emergence of alternative aesthetics and politics of being human, living on Earth, and sharing the planet with other human beings and species. The second is focused on the resistance to what Mbembe sees as epistemic hegemony, the temptation to reduce Earth and all life forms to a financial problem, and the accompanying drive to automate society. And finally, the third strategy is preoccupied with connecting the fight against racism to ideas of human interdependence, radical sharing, and universal inclusion (Mbembe 2021a: 27–28; Mbembe 2021b: 20–21, 41). And no matter how inviting these possible remedies may seem, the truth is, the complex problems brought about by the biopolitics of extraction and use are not likely to be solved by the power of words alone – tangible actions still need to be taken to embody the change.

This last strategy, aimed at maximizing universal equality and prosperity, as suggested by Mbembe, appears to be especially relevant when analyzing the interplay of pandemic and race, as it was precisely the lack, or even absence of human interdependence, radical sharing, and universal inclusion that has aggravated the existing structural racial inequality during the pandemic. The COVID-19 pandemic has only confirmed both the shared condition of social life and human interdependency, as well as the pervasive racial inequality that has largely contributed to the greater likelihood of dying for those who are racially marginalized and the greater actual number of deaths. In her brief yet well-formulated overview of state racism and state violence in the wake of the Black Lives Matter movement, political philosopher Myisha Cherry highlights the arbitrariness of state racism by arguing that all citizens are susceptible to the phenomenon of racialization. The state can reduce a particular group to a sub-race at any given time, and their delegation to that category and the violence directed at them, as a result, has a huge impact on all people, regardless of their skin color. However, Cherry sees this biopolitical condition not as a sign of impending doom but rather as an opportunity to solidify a new sort of solidarity that is born out of the realization of the inherent vulnerability that we all share as citizens, as each of us could be targeted and/or affected by state racism and state violence in other ways. Cherry does so by proposing the notion of *vulnerable solidarity* and offering two arguments in support of her cause. First, vulnerability is universal and powerful because it creates a stronger motivation to fight against injustice than emotionally driven responses stemming from empathy. Second, the notion of vulnerable solidarity acknowledges that every individual, despite his or her ostensibly secure status, is susceptible to attacks or any other state-inflicted harm: "Vulnerable solidarity opens up the bonds of trusts among 'vulnerable' groups, which may be difficult to do with groups defined by their supra- and sub-race identities. Instead of joining a cause because it has a direct impact on our social positioning now, people will join causes because they will know that all injustices have an impact on us all; if not directly, indirectly, if not now, in the future" (Cherry 2017: 360–361). Ultimately, such a perspective eliminates the need to identify with a particular vulnerable group and, at the same time, marks a radical shift in the very approach to thinking identity as such. A similar perspective is shared by Judith Butler, who claims that the pandemic has allowed us to understand shared vulnerability and interdependency – in a straightforward, corporeal way – by making us realize that we share both the air we breathe and the surfaces of the world. For her, the idea that being infectious and becoming infectious are interconnected is inseparable from the phenomenological experience of the pandemic. Consequently, this understanding upturns our usual sense of the bounded self, as it reveals humans as relational, interactive beings, while at the same time rejecting the ego-logical, self-interested foundations of ethics itself (Butler 2022: 11–12). It could be said to constitute the fourth, and perhaps the most promising – solidary – cure for the current necropolitical disease, whose existence is hard to deny after taking a closer look at the interplay between pandemic and race.

6 Concluding Remarks

Notwithstanding the widespread uproar against structural racial inequality and its ongoing long-term effects, the un(fore)seen circumstances brought about by the emerging COVID-19 virus, which rapidly caused a global pandemic, allowed for the intensification of the existing racial dynamics inherent to biopower. This manifested itself via the capitalization of healthcare and life itself, the replacement of the classic Foucauldian "making life or letting die" equation with the differentiation between lives to be saved and lives to be risked, or life in the factory vs. life of the factory debate, and the acceleration of slow deaths that merely exacerbated the existing racial inequality. And though numerous solutions have been offered that might help to combat the necropolitical effects of the COVID-19 pandemic on race, including decolonial, politico-economic, ecological, and solidary perspectives, the worldwide efforts to contain the pandemic often resulted only in furthering the existing racial inequality and reinforcing the existing necropolitical regimes of exclusion, largely based on the politics of extraction and use.

As the pandemic has largely withdrawn from the newspaper headlines and given way first to Russia's full-scale invasion of Ukraine and then to the Israel-Palestine conflict, one can finally see how the world has changed – or rather, how it has not changed at all. The anthropogenic climate change continues, radical political–economic transformations do not seem likely to be implemented on the planetary level anytime soon, and we are left aching for the solution to the age-old impasse of the biopolitics of extraction and use, which targets the most deprived and the most vulnerable, who are often racially marginalized, too. However, this necropolitical deadlock will not be resolved unless we reject the biopolitical logic, accept the understanding of humans as relational beings, and embrace the idea that everyone's life matters equally, regardless of race, which is used and abused to justify and maintain the global structural racial inequality by subjecting the world's populations to barely concealed categorization way too often.

References

Aburto, J. M., Tilstra, A. M., Floridi, G., Dowd, J. B. 2022. "Significant Impacts of the COVID-19 Pandemic on Race/Ethnic Differences in US Mortality," *PNAS*, 119(35), https://www.pnas.org/doi/epdf/10.1073/pnas.2205813119. Accessed 6 February 2024.

Agamben, G. 2021. *Where Are We Now? The Epidemic as Politics*, translated by V. Dani. London: Eris.

Ahmed, S. 2019. *What's the Use? On the Uses of Use*. Durham: Duke University Press.

Ayala-Colqui, J. 2020. "Viropolitics and Capitalistic Governmentality: On the Management of the Early 21st Century Pandemic," *Desde el Sur*, 12 (2): 377–395.

Ajana, B. 2021. "Immunitarianism: Defence and Sacrifice in the Politics of COVID-19", *HPLS*, 43: 25, https://link.springer.com/article/10.1007/s40656–021–00384–9. Accessed 6 February 2024.

Becker, G. S. 2007. "Health as Human Capital: Synthesis and Extensions," *Oxford Economic Papers* 59 (3): 379–410.

Berlant, L. 2007. "Slow Death (Sovereignty, Obesity, Lateral Agency)," *Critical Inquiry*, 33 (4): 754–780.

Breu, C. 2013. "Subject and Substance: The Limits of Biopolitics and the Status of Critique", *English Language Notes*, 51 (2): 45–60.

Boukalas, Ch. 2023. *Biosecurity, Economic Collapse, the State to Come: Political Power in the Pandemic and Beyond.* Oxon and New York: Routledge, https://doi.org/10.4324/9781003302988. Accessed 6 February 2024.

Butler, J. 2022. *What World Is This? A Pandemic Phenomenology.* New York: Columbia University Press.

Cherry, M. 2017. "State Racism, State Violence, and Vulnerable Solidarity," in N. Zack (ed.), *The Oxford Handbook on Philosophy and Race.* Oxford: Oxford University Press, 352–362.

Fassin, D. 2007. "Humanitarianism as a Politics of Life," *Public Culture* 19 (3): 499–520.

Feldman, J. M., Bassett, M. T. 2021. "Variation in COVID-19 Mortality in the US by Race and Ethnicity and Educational Attainment", *JAMA Network Open*, 4(11), https://jamanetwork.com/journals/jamanetworkopen/fullarticle/2786466. Accessed 6 February 2024.

Foucault, M. 2003. *Society Must Be Defended: Lectures at the College de France, 1975–1976*, translated by D. Macey. London: Picador.

Harvey, D. 2000. *Spaces of Hope.* Edinburgh: Edinburgh University Press.

Harvey, D. 2020. "We Need a Collective Response to the Collective Dilemma of Coronavirus", *Jacobin*, 20th April, 2020, https://jacobin.com/2020/04/david-harvey-coronavirus-pandemic-capital-economy. Accessed 6 February 2024.

Lorenzini, D. 2020. "Biopolitics in the Time of Coronavirus," *Critical Inquiry*, 47 (S2): S40–S45.

Lorenzini, D. 2024. "Rethinking biopolitics: COVID-19, differential vulnerabilities and biopolitical rights," *Journal of European Studies*, 54 (1): 27–41.

Mackenzie, C., Rogers, W., Dodds, S. 2014. "Introduction: What Is Vulnerability and Why Does It Matter for Moral Theory?", in Mackenzie, C. et al. (eds.). *Vulnerability: New Essays in Ethics and Feminist Philosophy.* Oxford and New York: Oxford University Press, 1–29.

Mbembe, A. 2017. *Critique of Black Reason.* Durham: Duke University Press.

Mbembe, A. 2019. *Necropolitics.* Durham: Duke University Press.

Mbembe, A. 2021a. "Futures of Life and Futures of Reason", *Public Culture*, 33 (1 (93)): 11–33.

Mbembe, A. 2021b. *Out of the Dark Night: Essays on Decolonization.* New York: Columbia University Press.

Mbembe, Achille. 2021c. "The Universal Right to Breathe," *Critical Inquiry*, 47 (S2): S59–S62, https://www.journals.uchicago.edu/doi/pdf/10.1086/711437. Accessed 6 February 2024.

Nancy, J.-L. 2021. "a Viral Exception," in Castrillón, F., Marchevsky, Th. (eds.) *Coronavirus, Psychoanalysis, and Philosophy: Conversations on Pandemics, Politics, and Society.* Oxon and New York: Routledge, 27.

Purnell, K. 2021. *Rethinking the Body in Global Politics: Bodies, Body Politics, and the Body Politic in a Time of Pandemic.* Oxon and New York: Routledge.

Randolph, N. 2021. "Making Live and Letting Die in COVID-19: The Biopolitics of Race, Space and Freedom," *Spectra* 8 (2): 7–18.

Richardson, E. T. 2020. *Epidemic Illusions: On the Coloniality of Global Public Health.* Cambridge, Mass: MIT Press.

Ristić, D., Marinković, D. 2022. "Biopolitics of Othering during the COVID-19 Pandemic." *Humanities and Social Sciences Communications*, 9 (49): 1–8, https://www.nature.com/articles/s41599-022-01435-7. Accessed 6 February 2024.

Sandset, T. 2021. "The Necropolitics of COVID-19: Race, class and slow death in an ongoing pandemic," *Global Public Health*, 16 (8–9): 1411–1423.

Schweiger, G. 2022. "Introduction: the Global and Social Consequences of the COVID-19 Pandemic – Ethical and Philosophical Reflections," in Schweiger, G. (ed.). *The Global and Social Consequences of the COVID-19 Pandemic: An Ethical and Philosophical Reflection.* Springer Nature (ebook), 1–16.

Silverio, S. A., De Backer, K., Dasgupta, T., Torres, O., Easter, A., Khazaezadeh, N. et al. 2022. "On Race and Ethnicity during a Global Pandemic: An 'Imperfect Mosaic' of Maternal and Child Health Services in Ethnically-Diverse South London, United Kingdom," *eClinicalMedicine* 48: 101433.

Solomos, J. 2021. "Race and Ethnicity in Pandemic Times," *Ethnic and Racial Studies* 44 (5): 719–734.

White, A. I. R. 2023.1 *Epidemic Orientalism: Race, Capital, and the Governance of Infectious Disease.* Stanford: Stanford University Press.

Žižek, S. 2020a. *PANDEMIC!: COVID-19 Shakes The World.* New York and London: OR Books.

Žižek, S. 2020b. *PANDEMIC! 2: Chronicles of a Time Lost.* New York and London: OR Books.

CHAPTER 4

Toward an Ethics of Dispossession: Philosophical Lessons from the Political Context of the COVID-19 Pandemic

J. D. Mininger

Abstract

This chapter considers how and why to mourn the worldwide mass deaths caused by COVID-19, first by examining Hannah Arendt's theory of dark times, in which, by virtue of common suffering, a contradictory experience follows that both unites and alienates. Second, the chapter considers forms of melancholy exhibited during the pandemic, which emerged to the detriment of the lesson that mourning, in contrast to melancholy, reveals and acknowledges social interdependence. Judith Butler's concept of dispossession is deployed to shape that lesson. Third, the chapter offers Michel Foucault's theorization of critique as a practice to accompany mourning in the act of identification with suffering if there is resistance to the systemic violence operative in ranking who can be counted and mourned from the COVID-19 pandemic's many victims.

Keywords

COVID-19 – dispossession – mourning – melancholy – critique

•••

> There are times in life when the question of knowing if one can think differently than one thinks, and perceive differently than one sees, is absolutely necessary if one is to go on looking and reflecting at all [...]. [W]hat is philosophy today – philosophical activity, I mean – if it is not the critical work that thought brings to bear on itself? In what does it consist, if not in the endeavor to know how

 | DOI:10.1163/9789004748187_006

> and to what extent it might be possible to think differently, instead of legitimating what is already known?
>
> MICHEL FOUCAULT, *The History of Sexuality, Vol. 2: The Use of Pleasure*

∵

Following some preliminary musings on what might be meant by the term "pandemic politics" and some contextual remarks made to introduce and frame the itinerary of the commentary to follow, this article addresses a cluster of discrete but closely related topics: dark times, melancholia, dispossession, and critique. Together they constitute a philosophically minded answer to the question of what lessons we should take from the recent COVID-19 pandemic in order to improve political approaches to forming and maintaining community and global collectivity(s).

1 Theorizing Pandemic Politics, and Other Related Tasks of Philosophy in Dark Times

Within the coordinates of a project on immunity and contagion that bears the COVID-19 pandemic in mind, the points in this chapter arose from the task of taking initial account of some of the notable contributions by continental philosophers on the pandemic and its many points of social, political, and psychological stress. This chapter takes the term "pandemic politics" as its privileged angle of approach. Admittedly, this is an imprecise and slippery phrase, though used intentionally. The question of what constitutes politics as such – at the very least in the form of the continued dissolution of the distinction between the private and the public realms – is something with which the pandemic context (among so many other contexts and phenomena that also do so) continually confronted us.

It is difficult enough to theorize politics without the word "pandemic" as a qualifier. Politics and the political require definition despite their ubiquitous usage. The latter term typically invokes Carl Schmitt's formulation in *The Concept of the Political* (2007) of the political as marked out by the friend/enemy distinction. There are some ways in which it would make good sense to ask after this meta-frame of the political under the conditions of the pandemic. At the very least, it would seem at first glance to submit well to the task of dividing up the world between friends and enemies. But the sticking place for this sort of pandemic politics, just as in Schmitt's own theory, is at the limit of who and/or what constitutes the category of an enemy. The question of (existentially) who counts as an enemy is at the heart of Schmitt's concerns about the political. Schmitt references the distinctive uses of the term *hostis,* in comparison to *inimicus*, citing their biblical (Greek) origins, the former aligned with a public enemy and the latter with a private enemy (Schmitt 2007: 28–29). Therefore, who counts as an enemy, in some instances, becomes a precursor to the pandemic-contextual question of who counts at all. For example, whose deaths are known and countable at all; whose lives are considered worthy of counting in COVID death numbers?

It may be impossible (and foolhardy) to separate certain political actions as "pandemic politics" and others as seemingly unrelated, while it is in the nature of the pandemic conditions to go to the core of who we are as political subjects and to question precisely that status. As part of the intellectual exercise of this academic chapter, I am approaching the role of philosophy as the task of thinking under the pandemic conditions; and of course, in thinking about the pandemic and the issues it raises in how we organize ourselves, both as societies, such as in the degradation of the social contract, and as individual subjects.

For this matter of philosophy's task vis-à-vis pandemic politics – that is, the task of thinking under pandemic conditions – the chapter draws from the platform of Martin Heidegger's well-known lecture course in Freiburg during the early 50s, *Was heisst Denken?*, and its translation into English: *What is Called Thinking?* (1976) The literal translation sounds awkward in English, but it is wonderfully illuminating for the various subtleties it offers, as Heidegger breaks the question down into four questions, including defining the word (e.g., what is the action of thinking and the meaning of the act of thinking?), placing it in the context of its engagement in the history of Western philosophy, asking after necessary preconditions for thinking to occur and inquiring about what sorts of situations and problems motivate us – even require us – to think.

Thinking under conditions of the pandemic requires most profoundly a recourse to Heidegger's aforementioned points about the necessary preconditions and motivations for thinking. These two areas of inquiry are, in notable respects, flipsides of the same coin. On the one side, there is the matter of what is needed to think; or, what does thinking call for? Hannah Arendt addresses this in "On Humanity in Dark Times: Thoughts about Lessing" (Arendt 1968: 9), where she writes: "We are still aware that thinking calls not only for intelligence and profundity but above all for courage." Arendt's *Men in Dark Times*, particularly the lead essay, "On Humanity in Dark Times: Thoughts about Lessing," not only considers an abstract answer to what thinking calls for (namely, courage) but also specifically provides her own courageous thought about what constitutes so-called dark times. It is the first key point offered here in theorizing pandemic politics.

On the other side of the coin is the matter of what it is that makes us think or what calls for thinking under our pandemic conditions. What calls for thinking? What *compels* us to think? Heidegger says, with almost comical predictably, that Being calls us to think. Being is the most thought-provoking motivator – "we take it to heart" (Heidegger 1976: 203), because it is the most fundamental. Setting aside Heidegger's sentimentality, in a basic sense here he is making a plea for pausing to pay attention to, and to care for, the singular fact of existence. He encourages the existential appreciation of "the presence of what is present" (Heidegger 1976: 235). This risks falling into the popular modern discourse of mindfulness. However, if this thinking vacuum is avoided, it leads to strong and focused thinking, in the sense of heightened self-reflexive thinking about the fact of existing and the many modes of living in which existence is expressed. In the pandemic context, this reflected thought of "the presence of what is present" (Heidegger 1976: 235) is won in contrast to the confrontation with the many who constitute an absence, as the many who died due to COVID-19 and whose lives we mourn not as a mere absence but specifically as a loss. It is this pandemic fact of death and the concomitant political significance of the need for mourning that is presented here as the second key point in theorizing pandemic politics.

Several volumes of scholarly research have already appeared in an attempt to address the philosophical and political questions that arose because of the COVID-19 pandemic. The recent volume edited by Pegah Mossleh, *Corona Phenomenon: Philosophical and Political Questions* (2022), addresses this by challenging a group of 25 scholars from Europe and North America to respond to one or more of the 60 questions posed in the book's Preface, categorized alternately as either "Philosophical Questions" or "Political Questions" (Mossleh 2022: xiv–xix).

Coronavirus, Psychoanalysis, and Philosophy: Conversations on Pandemics, Politics, and Society, edited by Fernando Castrillón and Thomas Marchevsky (2021), captures a mid-pandemic conversation among notable continental philosophers, such as Jean-Luc Nancy, Giorgio Agamben, Roberto Esposito, Sergio Benvenuto, and Julia Kristeva. The volume presents a good starting place for surveying many of the academic positions already staked out on this general topic. Most of these essays not otherwise explicitly about the insights of psychoanalysis are meant to address either terrain covered by Giorgio Agamben, or terrain populated by Agambenian concepts which these philosophers would like to re-sculpt: e.g. biopolitics, state of exception, naked life, and *homo sacer*. These are all important concepts in their own right, and in this pandemic context, the scholarly rejoinders to Agamben's provocations are equally valid and important. I have little commentary for that entire exchange. Of course, the biopolitical operations of a state limiting the freedom of a population via health regulations is, at least in the abstract, a serious issue and one to contend with. But Agamben's position at points almost reaches a reactionary conspiracy theory level, and the basic point made by numerous theorists is simply one that I would echo: yes, a "green pass" or its equivalent does limit individual and collective freedom; however, has not dying from COVID-19 limited it that much more radically? In other words, rather than retrace the issues of personal liberty and government overreach, I would prefer to resituate the coordinates of philosophizing about the pandemic to consider time – not temporality in the sense of timing, but more in line with historical time and what Hannah Arendt borrows from a Bertolt Brecht poem to call: "dark times" (Arendt 1968), such as in the phrase people utter when they wish to speak about the present as history: "what times we live in!" I refer here to "times" as a kind of Lacanian *Thing*, that is, a concept borne of immanent causality.

How can circumstances of suffering help illuminate the search for meaning? It is the overarching frame of Arendt's volume of essays titled *Men in Dark Times*, published in 1968, which, along with a lead essay that looks back to Lessing for inspiration, contains essays on the lives and work of Rosa Luxemburg, Karl Jaspers, Walter Benjamin, Isak Dinesen, Hermann Broch, and Bertolt Brecht, among others. While her use of "dark times" references the World Wars of the twentieth century, punctuated by the Holocaust, what she means by dark times is not simply an era full of monstrosities and disaster, but especially a time in which a particular function of politics is lost. What is lost is an enlightenmentish public realm where the affairs of citizens can be demonstrated and "a space of appearances in which they can show in deed and word, for better and worse, who they are and what they can do" (Arendt 1968: viii). Darkness arrives when "this light is extinguished by 'credibility gaps' and 'invisible government', by speech that does not disclose what is but sweeps it under the carpet, by exhortations, moral and otherwise, that, under the pretext of upholding old truths, degrade all truth to meaningless triviality" (Arendt 1068: viii). In this sense, dark times are when horrible things are happening, yet they are not fully politically visible – they are either covered up or explained away.

A fitting example is the handling of the pandemic in the United States by former President Trump and his administration. There surely is little detail that needs to be provided in support of this connecting point: Trump's statements during the pandemic were repeatedly about how the curve is flattening, or the numbers "aren't that bad," or the numbers are "fake news," and so forth. Another US-based example of the pandemic as dark times is noted by Fernando Castrillon and Thomas Marchesvky in the introductory essay to their edited volume(2021), where they point out that the United States:

> instead of *utilizing* the pandemic and concerns regarding biosecurity to extend its reach and introduce restrictive political measures that were unthinkable just a few months ago, the federal government has relinquished this opportunity so as to exert its power via an already overwhelming repressive apparatus – a long-standing feature of North American statecraft, as exemplified by the recent and blatant use of heavily armed federal Department of Homeland Security agents to violently crush mostly peaceful protests against the relentless police killings of African Americans.
>
> CASTRILLON AND MARCHESVKY 2021: 8

In this version of dark times, the supposed light is itself the bearer of a kind of political darkness. What happens within this broad stroke definition of dark times, explains Arendt, is the loss of *world* in the Heideggerian sense (Arendt 1968: ix). Arendt argues that "this in-between – much more than (as is often thought) men or even man – is today the object of greatest concern and the most obvious upheaval in almost all of the countries of the globe" (Arendt 1968: 4). In other words, according to Arendt, in dark times people experience an undoing of their social bonds. In the case of the pandemic, this is not only the perceived nature of the deterioration of social bonds but the physical–spatial relationships as well, due to isolation, most notably, among other things.

For example, consider the theorization of immunity as a mediating function between organism and environment: symbiosis is the rule, not the exception. Immunity participates in an ecosystem because the difference between self and non-self is fluid, dynamic, and relational. Immunity is not so much a defense response as a general cognitive capacity. It is precisely that capacity that Arendt points to as eroding in dark times. The interspaces of human subjects are lost, either as perceived or as otherwise really existing. This same phenomenon is treated well by Roberto Esposito in his article *Vitam instituere* (Castrillon and Marchevsky 2021: 87–88) under the formulation of the dissolution of symbolic ties.

Arendt points to a dangerous but important two-fold potential in the way in which people bond together in dark times, whether intentionally or inevitably: *fraternité* [brotherhood] and friendship. In dark times, a particular kind of human relationship and interaction develops, occasioned by common suffering. Arendt explains:

> humanity manifests itself in such brotherhood most frequently in "dark times." This kind of humanity actually becomes inevitable when the times become so extremely dark for certain groups of people that it is no longer up to them, their insight or choice, to withdraw from the world. Humanity in the form of fraternity invariably appears historically among persecuted peoples and enslaved groups [...]. This kind of humanity is the great privilege of pariah peoples.
>
> ARENDT 1968: 13

The pressure of persecution reduces "the interspace which we have called world" (Arendt 1968: 13) to nothing. In the extreme situation of dark times, "the pariahs of this world enjoy the great privilege of being unburdened by care for the world" (Arendt 1968: 14); or, they are simply worldless in the Heideggerian sense, literally with no immunity, no symbiosis, and no suitable relationship between self and world, or between organism and environment.

This *fraternité* occasioned by dark times, on one hand, produces warmth and bonds between those experiencing the common suffering. However, paradoxically, these circumstances also create worldlessness and a lack of connectivity with others, which immunity would otherwise provide. For the COVID-19 pandemic context, there is a (set of) particular relationship(s) in this regard. Rather than the consolidation of minority communities that happens via shared suffering, we witnessed a proliferation of these pariah relations within the pandemic context. In other words, everyone felt oppressed and seemed to belong to one or another fraternity. In the pandemic, we were all pseudo-pariahs. "Pseudo" because those truly in this category, those for whom "the times become so extremely dark [...] that it is no longer up to them, their insight or choice, to withdraw from the world" (Arendt 1968: 13), are the true witnesses to the dark times of the pandemic, for they are the ones who died. These are the pandemic pariahs truly "unburdened by care for the world" (Arendt 1968: 14).

2 Mourning and Melancholia in the COVID-19 Pandemic; or, toward an Ethics of Dispossession

As of September 29, 2022, the number of deaths due to COVID-19 is over 6.5 million. This is according to *The New York Times*, JHU CSSE COVID-19 Data, and "Our World in Data" (which, if to immediately invoke the unconscious, is a spectacularly and irreducibly biopolitical title for a data collection and management site). There have been over 1 million deaths in the United States, over half a million in India, nearly 700,000 in Brazil, approximately 150,000 in France, and the same in Germany. In Lithuania, one of the EU's smaller countries and home to less than 3 million residents, there have been 9,319 deaths due to COVID-19 as of the aforementioned date. Where I reside at the time of completing this chapter – Bulgaria – there have been 37,711 COVID-related deaths.

But this is not really the truth of the matter, is it? These are numbers – facts; they are truthful in their own way. But they are no doubt also incorrect in terms of how many actually died of COVID-19. No doubt there were so many more: unrecorded, unnoted, or uncounted. But the accuracy of the count is not the truth I mean here. While these numbers are "mind-boggling," as we often casually say, I do not wish to reference some form of sublime truth: an incalculability or ineffability or overwhelming power; or, to be more precisely Kantian about the category, I do not intend truth here as the subject's experience of what it cannot cognize or synthesize with the combination of imagination and reason. Admittedly, this is getting closer to the intended meaning.

If we ask these numbers – "our world in data" – to help us understand not merely how many but *who* these people are that died, we get still closer to my point of interest. In an article in *The Guardian*, Shirley Smith (2021) reports about a collaborative study by the Centers for Disease Control and Prevention (CDC), Imperial College London, Harvard University, Oxford University and the University of Cape Town, published in the journal *Pediatrics* back in October of 2021. From this study, we learn that "from April 2020 to June 30, 2021, in the US, more than 140,000 children under the age of 18 lost their mother, father, or grandparent who provided their housing, basic needs and daily care to the disease. The study reveals that COVID-19 is not only disproportionately killing adults from communities of colour, but the children in these communities are bearing the brunt of the aftershock of this 'hidden pandemic'" (Smith 2021). Not all people and communities were equally agile in adjusting to the social, psychological, and physiological stresses caused by many factors of the COVID-19 pandemic, including lifestyle changes caused by the requirements for precaution (e.g., quarantine), but first and foremost, the danger of the virus itself. Of course, the virus does not account for human differences, but our human social and political lives are structured by inequitable differentiations.

The truth about COVID-19-related deaths at stake in this inquiry is also a matter of a kind of accounting, but it is neither about the accuracy of the reckoning nor the impossibility of systematically and wholly understanding what we have reckoned. It is the pandemic fact of *mass death*, and the matter of how we have and have not acknowledged this mass death as loss, which I wish to comment upon. As an important aside, I wish to clearly state that private, personal, individual loss is very real, of course, and very truthful, and it deserves attention, too. This chapter limits its scope to considering mass death.

The political significance of acknowledging (or not acknowledging) mass death as loss resides to a great degree in the need for a process of mourning. In a 2020 interview, Judith Butler comments on her then-contemporaneous pandemic context, explaining that: "learning to mourn mass death means marking the loss of someone whose name you do not know, whose language you may not speak, who lives at an unbridgeable distance from where you live" (Butler 2020). When we mourn and mark death as loss in this way, the lesson exposed is that we are inextricably interdependent on others; our very existence requires others. In this context, the process of mourning admits not merely our own vulnerability but also our always already-entangled lives (with others) and the vulnerability of those others. Thus, the insights about interdependence, intersection, emergent theorizations of community, ethology, and transindividuality, which many others have thoughtfully considered in reflection upon the pandemic, I am merely reminding us about via some philosophical and psychoanalytic concepts.

I posit that the truth of COVID-19 mass death is the true political pole around which all points in pandemic politics ultimately turn, regardless of the heated tensions that arise surrounding supposed individual freedoms, rights, etc. Therefore, we must discuss the matter of addressing those deaths in the form of mourning for the sake of "collective ego health" or the health of the social body (or whatever). But we must also ask how we mourn the mass deaths of the pandemic as a productive opportunity to seek a politics and a mode of negotiating our collective living that accounts for truth not along axes of accurate/inaccurate or possible/impossible, but, rather, in a way that is consonant with the experience of having our radical global social interdependence exposed.

One excellent way that the question of how to mourn the mass death of the COVID-19 pandemic has been answered is by turning to lessons learned from Sophocles' *Antigone*. Among these lessons is the cultural importance of burial rites, as discussed by psychoanalyst Nestor Braunstein in "The Return of Antigone: Burial Rites in Pandemic Times" (Braunstein 2021: 66–75). The value of this approach to mourning is the insistence on understanding that, as Braunstein notes, burial rituals "make death a social event and not an individual avatar" (Castrillon and Marchevsky 2021: 72). But it is not enough to simply say: we need to bury, we need to acknowledge and mourn, we need to cry out, and so forth. For example, the act of wailing is an exceptional, important, and interesting form of mourning. But just as in explaining religious faith, we say, "kneel and you shall believe," the health (for lack of a better term) that one seeks for both subject and society through the process of mourning is only ever an effect of its own effects – it "is" only as it "does" and we merely name it afterward with a convenient title or conceptual place-holder. In other words, mourning is not a simple mechanism.

Mourning does, however, often conform to simple definitions. In "Mourning and Melancholia," Freud writes that "mourning is regularly the reaction to the loss of a loved person, or to the loss of some abstraction which has taken the place of one, such as one's country, liberty, and ideal, and so on" (Freud 1953: 243). Mourning, as Renata Salecl clarifies, "is the process of the separation from the object, which no longer exists" (Salecl 2004: 29). Through various attempts to test reality, the bereaved person detaches themselves from the lost object and, in an overly simplistic sense, accepts the loss as a loss.

Perhaps the most intriguing category from Freud's famous article is not mourning but melancholy, which Freud contrasts with what he refers to as normal mourning. If to be teleological about this in the sense of being therapeutic, the lesson from Freud is that mourning must attempt to avoid falling into melancholia, lest the grieving subject narcissistically turn that grief on itself with such results as traumatic repetition and a kind of paralysis of productive, transformative action. In other words, mourning must avoid melancholia lest the grieving subject becomes unable to move on, productively work through the loss, and live for themselves as opposed to living with the loss itself as the unconscious and absent center, conditioning their desires. Judith Butler explains the structure of melancholia in the following way: "I cannot live in a world in which the object I value is lost, or I cannot be the person who has lost what I value. I will destroy the world that reflects to me that which I have lost, or I will leave that world through recourse to fantasy. This form of denial would rather destroy reality, to hallucinate a preferred reality, than register the verdict of loss that reality has to deliver" (Butler 2021). Mourning seeks a way to mark loss by consciously and intentionally communicating (about) the loss. But if mourning falls into a kind of narcissistic melancholia, then it loses the insight that was to be won from mourning mass death in the pandemic context; namely, the crucial understanding of human existence as fundamentally interpenetrative, multiple, and irreducibly interdependent on one another and on the entirety of our environments.

Nowhere were the stakes of acknowledging the mass deaths of COVID-19 more apparent than in the Trump administration's refusal to mourn, and in many instances, this refusal came in the form of outright denial of loss. The inability to accept loss in any form is the distinguishing characteristic of Trump's individual character in the first place. He acted, and still acts, in the parlance of the pandemic, as if he were immune to lack. This particular point in which lack seems to be lacking is precisely one of the definitions Jacques Lacan provides for anxiety (see Lacan 2015), which is a discrete but related reaction to the loss of an object. As Renata Salecl explains, "anxiety signals a danger over the loss of the object, whereas melancholy appears as a solution to this, as the subject insists in identification with the lost object" (Salecl 2004: 30). Following Lacanian thinking, in not mourning the mass deaths with greater public and political acknowledgement, we effectively are denying lack as such, i.e., we seem to be abolishing desire. We experience but do not register a kind of loss of loss itself. But this sort of melancholic posture is, of course, not the abolishing of desire but rather simply the locating of a more particular form of jouissance. Allow me to suggest several notable illustrations from the pandemic of this melancholic mode in which we desperately try to fill the lack and maintain the frame of fantasy otherwise supporting that lack:

1. We saw a continuing intensification of the ever-desperate search for self-recognition and the fixing of static identities. For example, "Who were we for these people whose lives were taken by COVID-19?" "Who are the enemies who have tainted my nation, my community, my school, my home, and so forth with this virus?" Rather than accept the reality of the extraordinary interdependence we necessarily share with the lives of strangers, the opportunity for filling new potentials for regressive political ideologies, such as nationalism, religious fundamentalism, tribalism, and so on appeared.
2. We saw painful forms of jouissance, such as new levels of alcoholism, hipster trends, such as "sourdough bread-baking" on Instagram, and enhanced lives as avatars on social media. Or, the example of rushing to Netflix as a form of self-anaesthetizing, which, on one hand, deflects reality, but on the other hand, redraws reality, as all storytelling ultimately does (or can do).
3. In the face of mass death, we saw an expansion of the symbolic importance of self-improvement during lockdown: "What did you do to improve yourself during quarantine?" "Every crisis is an opportunity, right? So, how can our business use the pandemic to learn new tricks, cross previously unbridgeable thresholds, and make ourselves [supposedly] better?" This particular melancholic posture turns out to be just one more baroque variation on the marriage between capitalism and

progress that, for example, Karl Marx theorized so poignantly in the *Grundrisse* in the 1850s.

Melancholy is one clear reaction to the COVID-19 mass deaths. Perhaps it is the most notable and prevalent response. However, like the good Saussurian sign that it is, melancholy's mutually constitutive partner in lexical value, mourning, also deserves attention – since, lest the picture be unfaithfully painted, there is certainly positive and reflective and important grieving that has taken place with respect to the mass deaths of COVID-19.

There are at least several important lessons to learn from mourning as a kind of political act in the context of and as a response to the COVID-19 pandemic and its mass deaths, all of which can be categorized under the umbrella term of vulnerability. Vulnerability is, ultimately, what is acknowledged in the act of mourning. While vulnerability in this context obviously refers to the potential for perceived physical harm, even and especially death, we can also follow Judith Butler in her expansion of the understanding of this term. She explains that "vulnerability is not just the condition of being potentially harmed by another. It names the porous and interdependent character of our bodily and social lives" (Butler 2020). Butler's concept of vulnerability aligns well with Spinoza's doctrine of mind-body parallelism: minds and bodies alike are treated as finite modes of a non-transcendent unique Substance, identified as God (or Nature). Our bodies are immanent to our environments, just as we affect and are affected by other bodies. In Butler's sense, in this context, our vulnerability is exposure to others' bodies (and not just human bodies): "to their gaze, their touch, their violence" (Lloyd 2008: 94).

In the act of mourning, we find some of our fundamental desires and commitments exposed, or so Butler suggests. She crucially describes the revelations of the interdependence of bodies that arise from grief and mourning as belonging to forms of dispossession (Lloyd 2008: 94). What she means by this term is that we are dispossessed "when loss occurs, that is, 'I think I have lost "you" only to discover that "I" have gone missing as well'" (Lloyd 2008: 94). As Maya Lloyd describes it, "loss reveals the subject's dependence on an other for its own sense of self and thus for its continued existence" (Lloyd 2008: 94). The dispossession that Butler describes is both epistemological in the sense that a condition is exposed to us by loss, namely, shared physical dependence. But that shared dependence is also a transformation of sorts in the self: I am no longer what I was, due not only to corporal porosity but also the shared social interdependence. In mourning, we (re)discover our dependence on other bodies and minds for a sense of self. Thus, according to Butler's concept, mourning is not just the act of ego health, not merely an affirmation of human vulnerability; but it is, as Lloyd contends of Butler's work, also an "opportunity for rethinking politics, and particularly international politics, in a less aggressive, more ethical mode" (Lloyd 2008: 93).

But, as the pandemic demonstrated time and again, many prefer to deny human vulnerability. This often manifests in onerous ways, most notably when it is deemed that "not all human lives are [...] worthy of grief" (Lloyd 2008: 94). To be inoculated against the normative systemic violence operative in ranking who can be mourned – that would be immunity worthy of the term. Thus, another key valence of Butler's concept of vulnerability is that it names not just a potential for harm and even death but "the greater likelihood of dying, understood as the fatal consequence of a pervasive social inequality" (Butler 2020). In this sense, the animating question here – how shall we mourn the COVID mass deaths – is not a practical matter of determining a set of "how to" instructions; instead, it is an ethical inquiry that invites the questions: whose lives may be mourned, and what makes for a grievable life? (Butler 2004: 20).

3 Dispossession as a Mode of Critique

While we might pose this inquiry about political life in general, irrespective of some particular era, the pandemic context has particular coordinates that help frame the following question: how can we be inoculated against the systemic and normative violence operative during a pandemic time, which ranks who can be counted among the dead, whose lives are grievable, who is in fact mourned, and how they are counted – let alone how their deaths are grieved and mourned as lives lost?

Answers should begin with a return to the matter of mourning itself. Whether it can fairly be articulated as a kind of inoculation, one initial answer to the question of how we seek to immunize ourselves against the normative violence inherent in the operation of power that ranks who can be mourned and how, is that the mourning process itself must be constituted by a two-fold movement: "identification with suffering must also include a certain critical reflexivity about the operations of this normative violence" (Lloyd 2008: 94). In "Violence, Mourning, and Politics," Judith Butler locates this critical reflexivity in the following passage:

> To grieve, and to make grief itself into a resource for politics, is not to be resigned to inaction, but it may be understood as the slow process by which we develop a point of identification with suffering itself. The disorientation of grief – "Who have I become?" or, indeed, "What is left of

> me?" "What is it in the Other that I have lost?" – posits the "I" in the mode of unknowingness. But this can be a point of departure for a new understanding if the narcissistic preoccupation of melancholia can be moved into a consideration of the vulnerability of others. Then we might *critically evaluate* and *oppose* the conditions under which certain human lives are more vulnerable than others, and thus certain human lives are more grievable than others. From where might a principle emerge by which we vow to protect others from the kinds of violence we have suffered, if not from an apprehension of a common human vulnerability?
>
> BUTLER 2004: 30, my emphases

This critical practice of evaluation is crucial if there is to be opposition to the normative violence that privileges some lives over others. The practice of critique noted by Butler must accompany mourning's work of identification with the suffering of a vulnerable community to which one belongs through the "porous and interdependent character of our bodily and social lives" (Butler 2020), yet through those who remain unknown in the simplistic sense of not individually recognized and remembered.

What is this critical activity, this critical reflexivity? While this is hardly the only conceptual vehicle for moving forward with a fitting answer to this question, Michel Foucault's theorization of critique is one important version of how we can understand and assess this vital critical reflexivity that must accompany mourning as its inoculatory bodyguard.

Foucault offers commentary on the concept, action, and ethos of critique in numerous places in his many books and lectures, and while there is certainly a strong continuity in these multiple treatments, it is not a systematically articulated concept. Nevertheless, there is one lecture from which to draw significant statements on the topic, a talk delivered to the French Society of Philosophy in May 1978, simply titled: "What is Critique?" This particular title lines up with a pattern in certain texts and lectures of straightforward "what questions" that utilize the inquiry structure whereby the subject to be specifically defined is replaced by the question "what": for example, What is an Author? What is Revolution? What is Enlightenment? No doubt, the simplicity of the posed question is used by contrast to ultimately underscore the complexity of the very act in these essays of inquiring into what it means to offer a definition as such in the first place and what the stakes of such acts of definition hold for matters of truth and the discourses and subjects made and maintained by these regimes of definitional truths. But in this case, in "What is Critique?" the title is no doubt also a distinct reference to the 1784 text written by Immanuel Kant in response to the question posed by Johann

Friedrich Zoellner in December of 1783 in the *Berlinische Monatsschrift*: "what is enlightenment?" Kant's well-known little text, "An Answer to the Question: 'What is Enlightenment?'", was an intellectual preoccupation (of sorts) for Foucault over the final 6 or 7 years of his life. The concept of critique that Foucault manages in the "What is Critique?" lecture emerges precisely from his consideration of the Kantian provocation about what constitutes enlightenment.

Lest we get sidetracked by cataloguing the varying interpretations of Kant's text about enlightenment (cf. Schmidt 1996), suffice it to explain briefly that arguably what Foucault prizes most in Kant's short text is that rather than a historically minded evaluation of an era or a movement or even a discourse, Kant outlines a generic critical procedure of enlightenment whereby the subject ultimately reinvents itself by making its way out of its "self-incurred immaturity" (1991). The critical attitude at work here involves discovering and showing that one's immaturity (in German: *Unmündigkeit*) is self-incurred; that is to say, it is contingently constructed – "it involves showing that we have been formed out of contingencies" (Tirkkonen 2018: 213). Thus, enlightenment helps us understand "not who we really are", but "that we do not have to be the same as before" (Tirkkonen 2018: 213). As regards the relationship between enlightenment and the term critique, in several different texts, Foucault argues for the essential continuity between Kant's critical enterprise (i.e., the three critiques) and the process of enlightenment. Though they are certainly not synonymous or fully transparent to one another, they "complement each other," claims Foucault in the opening two lectures of the 1982–83 lecture series dedicated to revisiting the Kantian enlightenment text (Foucault 2010: 31). Another important point Foucault gleans from Kant's text is an insistence that Kant's enlightenment procedure is both an individual and collective attitude. He confirms that social development must surely be plural and must surely be animated by a "we" – even if that "we" has no pre- or prior-established homogeneous identity.

Foucault's notion of critique emerges from the Kantian enlightenment context, as a political condition for critique that involves the potential for self-transformation. But Foucault also stretches beyond the strict Kantian context to see in this critical attitude of enlightenment an ethos that, in its potentiality and open-ended direction, might very well displace the Kantian notion of critique as "the attempt to investigate the requirements of the possibility of concrete philosophical endeavors" (Hammermeister 2002: 24), i.e., self-limitation on the basis of investigating the current conditions of one's activities. Of these potentially lofty (perhaps even utopian) political dimensions, Foucault writes:

> I mean an analysis that relates to what we are willing to accept in our world, to accept, to refuse, and to change, both in ourselves and in our circumstances. In sum, it is a question of searching for *another kind of critical philosophy*. Not a philosophy that seeks to determine the conditions and the limits of our possible knowledge of the object, but a critical philosophy that seeks the conditions and the indefinite possibilities of transforming the subject, of transforming ourselves.
>
> FOUCAULT 1993: 224, my emphasis

This indistinct critical philosophy of indefinite possibilities accompanies Foucault's theorization of critique as its virtual possibility. But Foucault also applies actualized actions to the ethos of critique, for it is also ultimately meant (sincerely) as a practical attitude – one that Foucault will even suggest is a virtue. "I would therefore propose," says Foucault in "What is Critique?", "as a very first definition of critique, this general characterization: the art of not being governed quite so much" (Foucault 2007: 45). Foucault locates this critical attitude within the historical dimension of the governmentalization of both society and individuals. Thus, for Foucault, the heart of the matter is not just mere resistance to the power dynamics of present governance of self and others, but also specifically the question: "How not to be governed *like that*, by that, in the name of those principles, with such and such an objective in mind and by means of such procedures, not like that, not for that, not by them" (Foucault 2007: 44). As we see here, much like with the example of "example," critique will depend on its objects for shape and recognition. However, as Foucault insists, critique is not equivalent to resistance, revolution, or even judgment. It isn't so – because critique is conceived here as an infinite and ongoing task: a constant practice of concrete sets of actions. Foucault positions critique beyond (in the sense, again, of inequivalence, not of irrelevance towards) being consistent about one's views (in the sense of critical judgments) and also beyond the sense Hannah Arendt gives to critique as the act of providing a foundation for the possibility of agreement. In subtle contrast – and in a move that is not far removed from the definition that Kant provided – Foucault will understand that the core of critique implicates the intertwining relations of truth, power, and the subject. He writes:

> I will say that critique is the movement by which the subject gives himself the right to question truth on its effects of power and question power on its discourses of truth. Well, then!: critique will be the art of voluntary insubordination, that of reflected intractability. Critique would essen-

> tially insure the desubjugation of the subject in the context of what we could call, in a word, the politics of truth.
>
> FOUCAULT 2007: 47

According to Foucault, critique means to throw the very frame of evaluation itself into relief and to illuminate how our epistemological certainties ultimately exclude other possible orderings. Critique means to question the limits of our surest ways of knowing. But precisely because of these dramatic philosophical and rhetorical turns, it is important to note that critique should, therefore, arise where a crisis plainly already exists in our epistemological fabric. For the pandemic context, I posit that this crisis is located in the notion of the self (or, put differently, life) as solitary and sovereign in relation to the COVID-19 virus, or, put differently, a crisis the result of which is that our "selves" are restrictedly understood as mere COVID crisis vessels. This fully inverts the immunity concept, which favors notions of interdependence, entangled life, and a sort of "ethology" in the sense that Deleuze theorizes the term in the essay "Spinoza and Us" (Deleuze 1988).

In the movement of critique, how do we move from understanding reasons for consenting to demand to form those for ourselves, then to transforming ourselves while producing them (and then perhaps risking the whole frame of reason as such)? In the context of this question, Foucault has insisted on the central impetus for critique: "how not to be governed *like that*" (Butler 2002: 9). The art of not being governed quite so much, as a constant practice and concrete action, shot-through as it is with reflection, is what aligns the concept of critique with virtue. Critique is potentially virtuous because it can be – it really must be – a constant relationship of caring for the self and others. Thus, it is a virtue that critique is also and always an ongoing task aimed at questioning all forms of domination. Virtue is more than an attitude or practice; it is a dynamic relation to norms, not just following rules or laws (Butler 2002: 6).

We might ask at this point, along with Butler in her "What is Critique? An Essay on Foucault's Virtue" (2002), how does self-transformation become a part of this? How is that (Kantian enlightenment-tinged) part of critique related to virtue? Foucault draws strongly from the example of obedience, surely influenced in this choice by the commitment to reading the Kantian enlightenment text. He differentiates in the predictable but highly productive way between command-based ethics and ethical practices of self-formation, drawing the line in the example of obedience between the virtue of obedience as such – reflected, practiced, and intended – and uncritical obedience to authority.

How can we translate this movement of critique, of "voluntary insubordination" (Foucault 2007: 47), into the context of pandemic politics? At the very least, we object to what we noted at the start: the imposition of the power of how we count lives, its costs, how it is done, and how such counting is administered. The politics of truth here and the stakes of critique now return to these key questions: who counts as a person? Who deserves to be protected? Who can be protected? What can I be? What can an "I" be under contemporary conditions?

In pursuit of this line of critique, we bump up against the point that "rationalization meets its limits in what Foucault calls in *What is Critique?* 'desubjugation'" (Butler 2002: 15). The will of critique (if such a desire can be defined) is always the will not be governed *thusly*, that is to say, as a particular, qualified, subjectivized subject.

To be dispossessed, to accept immunity as interdependence instead of defense, means that certain critical reflexivity must accompany mourning in the form of critique about the operations of power surrounding pandemic politics; but, as critique in this Foucauldian sense, the frame of reference can be questioned, since it risks the deformation and/or decentering of the political subject, who occupies a position that does not and cannot guarantee the rules and order in advance: "who will be a subject here?" and "what will count as life"? (Butler 2002: 20)

References

Arendt, H. 1968. *Men in Dark Times*. New York: Harcourt, Brace & World, Inc.

Braunstein, N. 2021. "The Return of Antigone: Burial Rites in Pandemic Times", in Castrillón, F. and Marchevsky, T. (eds.). *Coronavirus, Psychoanalysis, and Philosophy: Conversations on Pandemics, Politics, and Society*. London: Routledge, 66–75.

Butler, J. 2002. "What is Critique? An Essay on Foucault's Virtue", in Ingram, D. (ed.). *The Political: Readings in Continental Philosophy*. London: Basil Blackwell.

Butler, J. 2004. *Precarious Life*. New York: Verso.

Butler, J. 2020. "Judith Butler: Mourning is a Political Act Amid the Pandemic and Its Disparities. Interview with George Yancy". Published in Truthout. April 30, 2020, https://truthout.org/articles/judith-butler-mourning-is-a-political-act-amid-the-pandemic-and-its-disparities/. Accessed 2 February 2024.

Butler, J. 2021. "Why Donald Trump will never admit defeat", *The Guardian*, January 20.

Castrillón, F. and Marchevsky, T. (eds.). 2021. *Coronavirus, Psychoanalysis, and Philosophy: Conversations on Pandemics, Politics, and Society*. London: Routledge.

Deleuze, G. 1988. "Spinoza and Us", in *Spinoza: Practical Philosophy*, translated by R. Hurley. San Francisco: City Lights Books.

Esposito, R. 2021. "Vitam Instituere", in Castrillón, F. and Marchevsky, T. (eds.). *Coronavirus, Psychoanalysis, and Philosophy: Conversations on Pandemics, Politics, and Society*. London: Routledge, 87–88.

Foucault, M. 1993. "About the Beginning of the Hermeneutics of the Self: Two Lectures at Dartmouth", *Political Theory* 21 (2): 198–227.

Foucault, M. 2007. "What is Critique?", in *The Politics of Truth*. New York: Semiotexte.

Foucault, M. 2010. *The Government of Self and Others: Lectures at the Collège de France 1982–1983*. London: Palgrave MacMillan.

Freud, S. 1953. "Mourning and Melancholia", in *The Standard Edition of the Complete Psychological Works of Sigmund Freud*, vol. 14, translated and edited by J. Strachey. London: Hogarth Press.

Hammermeister, K. 2002. *The German Aesthetic Tradition*. Cambridge: Cambridge University Press.

Heidegger, M. 1976. *What is Called Thinking?* Translated by J. G. Gray. Reprint Edition. New York: Harper Perennial.

Kant, I. 1991. "An Answer to the Question 'What is Enlightenment?'", in *Political Writings*, edited by H. S. Reiss, translated by H. B. Nisbet. Cambridge: Cambridge Press.

Lacan, J. 2015. *Anxiety: The Seminar of Jacques Lacan. Book X*, translated by A. R. Price. Cambridge: Polity Press.

Lloyd, M. 2008. "Towards a Cultural Politics of Vulnerability: Precarious Lives and Ungrievable Deaths," in Carver and Chambers (eds.). *Judith Butler's Precarious Politics: Critical Encounters*. London and New York: Routledge, 92–141.

Mossleh, P., ed. 2022. *Corona Phenomenon: Philosophical and Political Questions*. Brill: Leiden and Boston.

Salecl, R. 2004. *On Anxiety*. London: Routledge.

Schmidt, J. 1996. *What Is Enlightenment?: Eighteenth-Century Answers and Twentieth-Century Questions*. Berkeley: University of California Press.

Schmitt, C. 2007. *The Concept of the Political*. Expanded edition. Chicago: The University of Chicago Press.

Smith, S. 2021. "More than 140,000 US children lost a parent or caregiver to COVID, study finds", *The Guardian*, 7 October.

Tirkkonen, S. 2018. *Experience in Michel Foucault's Philosophy*. Helsinki: Unigrafia.

PART 2

Post-pandemic Biopolitics: Subjectivities, Spatialities, Temporalities

CHAPTER 5

The Death of Man: the Post-pandemic Condition?

Denis Petrina

Abstract

This chapter is inspired by Foucault's remark on "the death of man" as reified by the recent COVID-19 pandemic. Philosophical reflection on the pandemic has mostly come from the areas of biopolitics and posthumanism, and in this respect, the chapter seeks to continue this crucial dialogue by drawing on Foucault's intellectual legacy and arguing that Foucault (as a thinker of epidemics, biopolitics, and, at least implicitly, posthumanism) makes a significant contribution to the field of what I call in this chapter philosophical "post-pandemic studies." The first section, which focuses on the body, moves away from traditional interpretations of Foucault's theorization of the body in the paradigm of productivity and pragmatics and, largely through engagement with early Foucault's works and post-pandemic thinkers, emphasizes the overlooked dimension of the body in Foucault – namely, its openness, vulnerability, and epistemological obscurity. The second section re-examines Foucault's biopolitics in the context of pandemic management, revealing that Foucauldian biopolitics has always been "more-than-human" rather than merely human. Finally, the third section is devoted to the "genealogy of the post-pandemic subject," which problematizes the humanist category of the subject and proposes, as an alternative, techniques of the self that would enable the epistemological death of the human and the birth of the posthuman.

Keywords

biopolitics – Foucault – the death of man – techniques of the self – posthumanism

1 First Fragments of Post-pandemic Genealogy

The final lines of "The Order of Things" are considered one of Foucault's most enigmatic and thus perplexing and provocative words:

 | DOI:10.1163/9789004748187_007

> One can certainly wager that man would be erased, like a face drawn in sand at the edge of the sea.
>
> 1970: 387

The words are both frightening and puzzling: what exactly does Foucault mean here by the swift, wave-like erasure of man of which he speaks so nonchalantly? What implications does it have for us as humankind? And, if taken literally, or at least with the necessary degree of seriousness – how, when, and why will this happen? The COVID-19 pandemic, due to its magnitude, intensity, and highly destructive nature, prompted us to ask similar questions, which, although they had different implications, revolved around the same idea – the death of man. The pandemic brought the painful subject of human mortality to the forefront: the deadly virus did not "show favoritism" or discriminate, claiming countless lives across all demographics. And while certain populations were inherently more vulnerable to the virus, no one could declare themselves safe.

The literal demise of man (*qua* humanity) did not occur – for better or worse. Nevertheless, I will argue that the onset and arduous duration of the pandemic has called into question a more subtle and nuanced understanding of the death of man of which Foucault spoke almost prophetically in 1966 – that of the *epistemological* nature. In other words, it was an invitation (albeit a harsh one) for us to radically reconsider the position of human in the sphere of knowledge. As Bratton aptly notes, COVID-19 exposed the crisis of philosophy, attested to its failure of the pandemic's test (2021: 10). Indeed, the pandemic has shaken our seemingly solid foundation of knowledge, raising questions about the conceptual tools by which we navigate the world. What is the human? What is the body? What is health? What is the world? – are just a few of the critical questions we were left with during – and even after – the pandemic. This is borne out by an increasingly growing corpus of posthuman "post/pandemic studies" research (e.g. Bratton (2021), Hayles (2021), Newman & Topuzovski (2021) that underscores the urgent need to demolish the ontological, epistemological, and ethical pedestal upon which humans have placed themselves. Posthumanism, especially in light of the recent pandemic, emphasizes the actual and potential limitations of existing human-centered epistemological regimes and calls for novel and alternative categories, frameworks, and perspectives that transcend conceptually claustrophobic humanist epistemes.

Foucault (even though he is not usually labeled a posthuman thinker) seems like a perfect contender for this quest for a number of reasons. The first and most obvious reason is the increased scholarly interest (including posthumanists') in Foucault's writings following the outbreak of the pandemic.[1] Foucault's detailed and committed engagement with the transhistorical subject of the epidemics as well as its contextualization within power mechanics and dynamics (the most seminal works being the lecture series "Society Must Be Defended" and "Security, Territory, Population") provided a crucial conceptual framework for understanding the COVID-19 pandemic. Second, as Sonja van Wichelen has argued, Foucault "conveyed the embryonic frameworks of biopolitics" (161), which, although primarily concerned with the government of the "a species of people" (Foucault 2009: 105), have a strong posthuman potential. This chapter will show how Foucault's less popular and less articulated conceptualizations of biopolitics, particularly through his notion of the "milieu," redefine the status of the human in the biopolitical field.

Ultimately, Foucault's theoretical framework of genealogy, through its historicization (and consequent problematization) of the category of the subject, serves as a handy methodological tool to expose the conceptual fissures within the theoretically contingent category of the human. The pandemic has raised pressing questions about our identity, agency, and autonomy as humans, culminating in the question of what kind of post-pandemic subject will emerge. In my attempt to provide a tentative answer to this query, I will draw on Stefan Herbrecheter's application of Foucauldian critical genealogy to posthumanism to sketch the contours of the figure of the post-pandemic posthuman whose blurred conceptual silhouette has been brought to light by the COVID-19 pandemic.

While this chapter is structured around the core of Foucault's theoretical insights, it reflects on them not only *with* but also *beyond* Foucault. Thus, I will refer to other thinkers' ideas that either resonate with or extend Foucauldian formulations (particularly from the field of posthuman and post-pandemic studies). In doing so, I intend to demonstrate how the Foucauldian project of critical post-anthropology, centered on the idea of the "death of man," moves beyond the traditional theoretical trajectories of re/reading Foucault. Such a reading offers insights into what might metaphorically be called "contagious theory," which, instead of explaining, structuring, assembling, and curating, renounces its organic and purist ambitions and digresses, mutates, and transforms from within, thus creating new contaminated infrastructures of meaning.

---

1 For example, the compendium of texts entitled "Coronavirus and philosophers" opens with an excerpt from Foucault's book "Discipline and Punish: The Birth of the Prison" on the governance of lepers and the plague.

2 The (Epistemological) Symptomatology of the Human Body

Disease, illness, and sickness are inescapably bodily events. The contraction of a virus signifies the abrupt manifestation of the biological within the horizon of the existential, acting as a poignant reminder that *cogito*, subjectivity and agency, are limited by their corporeal situatedness; indeed, illness, in its own dramatic way, elucidates the inherently vulnerable materiality and fragile relationality of our living bodies, their precarious openness to a variety of others, our bodies' entanglement with the world's organic and inorganic parts, which at times, especially in the case of the disease, become virtually inseparable. Disease, falsely construed as pathology, as Foucault's teacher, Georges Canguilhem aptly observes, is nothing more than nature's way of establishing its own equilibrium, a deviation from the established biological path, a dysfunction urgently needed for the dynamic functionality and operation of the living body (1991: 41).

It may seem that this prologue correlates poorly with the Foucauldian conceptualization of the body, which is conventionally perceived in terms of social constructivism and political economy. In the disciplinary schema (the most commonly applied conceptual framework when reconstructing Foucault's notion of the body), as Protevi rightly notes, the body is typically associated with the machine due to its kinetic-mechanical nature and productive capacities. In biopolitical terms, the body appears as an anatomic apparatus fueled by "a composition of forces" that biopower, in its attempt to make use of the body, seeks to extract, manipulate, and exploit (Protevi 2015: 52). Nevertheless, the body is never easily and readily accessible to biopower: the operation, of which Foucault speaks as reductionist in "Discipline and Punish," which turns the body into "political force" and the assemblage and organization of living bodies into "political anatomy" (1995: 221), appears to mask another problem pertaining to the body – its ambivalent epistemological status (which was only reinforced during the pandemic, as we faced the incommunicable biological stratum of our bodies).

Thus, in order to explore the problem of the (diseased) body better, I move away from the pragmatist understanding of the body, which focuses on the effects the body produces, and instead discuss the body beyond the "semiotechniques" and "ideological codes" (Foucault 1995: 255) that power imposes on it. In "The Birth of the Clinic," when describing the doctor's gaze as a method of knowing the body, Foucault writes that it "is directed initially not towards that concrete body, that visible whole, that positive plenitude that faces him (…) but towards intervals in nature, lacunae, distances" (2003: 8). The pan-medicalization of virtually all spheres of life during the pandemic led us to acquire the medical optics described by Foucault for our own bodies. This internalized "doctor's gaze" made us see these "intervals, lacunae, distances" in our and other bodies, confronted with the risk of contracting a potentially lethal virus, and made us realize what fragile constructs our bodies are. The pandemic performed the reversal of the neoliberal myth of the omnipotent, perfectly functioning, unbreakable body; the repertoire of the necessary pandemic semio-techniques of the body (such as washing hands, wearing masks, and social distancing, to name a few) emphasized the fact that the body is heavily dependent on external prostheses to survive – especially in such a critical situation as a global epidemic. Most importantly, the threatening omnipresence of the virus brought *negative* potentiality – the potentiality of sickness, debilitation, or even death – to the fore.

In her article on COVID-19 as an anti-ableist experiment, Jurga Jonutytė reframes the problem of the traditional epistemologies of the body, emphasizing its opacity and obscurity (of which Foucault spoke so vividly), which dominant regimes of power tend to conceal. Following the feminist theorist of disability Margrit Shildrick, she questions the autonomy of the subject, asking important questions about whether the subject is in control of its own body, whether the body, placed in a neoliberal context, is a *possession* of the subject, its instrumentalized object; ultimately, whether the fact of embodiment is an epistemological alibi that proves the stable, singular, and identical nature of the human agency. The body is situated in the world as *openness to it* and is thus entangled with many other bodies – human and non-human, organic and inorganic, interrelated and interdependent, those in accordance with it, and, conversely, those that could hinder or harm each other. This entanglement blurs the seemingly fixed and unquestionable boundaries between the bodies, which, in this configuration, inevitably affect and are affected by each other. "After the limits start to fluctuate and, at the same time, to renew, the personal relation to the own body starts to change. The human body, including my own, becomes similar to any other piece of nature: not fully knowable, not explainable, but in all cases – multiple," she writes (Jonutytė 2022: 182).

When limits, boundaries, and frontiers become blurred, the human subject is struck by anxiety. On the one hand, anxiety is a psychosomatic response to uncanny uncertainty; once the initial panic over the outbreak of the pandemic subsided, it turned into a deadly paralyzing anxiety because the world as it was then became devoid of any meaning and purpose of the world as it had been before. On the other hand, however, as Jonutytė insightfully points out, there is a deeper, more disturbing, and therefore requiring more examination layer of anxiety, which she calls "existential anxiety": "a concern usually related to the questions about human race, human life, and its finitude, the questions of security and/or precarity of human body" (Ibid.: 176). To be a body means to be precarious, vulnerable, and susceptible to changes whose outcome can never be known in advance. The anxiety of being sick, ill, weak, and/or wounded (which, as Canguilhem argues, are relative, not absolute states) stems from our encounter with the inherently dark, opaque, and obscure nature of our bodies, which are never an organic given, but rather, in constant flux, in processual and unpredictable becomings – always and inevitably potentially accompanied by *un*becomings.

Gilles Deleuze and Félix Guattari, in their oeuvre *Anti-Oedipus* (the preface of which was written by Foucault), greatly expand and elaborate on the Foucauldian machinic concept of the body, offering a compelling detour from the intertwining theoretical trajectory of "body/power." For them, the machine is an ontological mode of affective entanglement that is not exclusive to humans or even living beings in general: "producing-machines, desiring-machines everywhere, schizophrenic machines, all species of life: the self and the non-self, outside and inside," they write (2000: 9). More surprising, however, is their formulation of the function of the machines, which, according to them, "work only when they break down and by continually breaking down" (Ibid.: 8). The operation of breaking down designates the limits of the body of which Jonutytė speaks, the ultimate being what Deleuze and Guattari call the "body without organs": the "decoded flows, at the limits of the codes and the territorialities [...] the absolute limit" (Ibid.: 170). To paraphrase, the "body without organs" is the body stripped of all cultural, social, economic, and political codes, of the organs on which the living body depends, the body whose intensity is 0 (Ibid.: 21), the unproductive, unrepresentative, unsignified, and unsubjugated body: liminal impotence.

Contextualized within the pandemic, the body without organs is the conceptual prototype of the sick body. The bodies of schizophrenics, drug addicts, and hypochondriacs come closest to the dangerous limits of the body without organs, which brings about total dissociation, dissolution, and ultimately, disintegration (Markula 2006: 38). Just as the body without organs denotes the meta/physical limits of the body, the sick body problematizes the naively celebrated potentiality of the human body, reminding us of the inversion of potentiality – impotence, absence of power, existential precariousness, and impossible limitations. The sick body reverses the famous Spinoza's formulation of "what the body can do," illuminating the shadowy and often hidden realm of the body's incapacity and impotence, exposing deeply rooted angst that arises from having a mortal and thus extremely vulnerable body.

The possibility of a radical shift – from a "healthy," well-functioning body to a suddenly impotent body – is conditioned by the fluctuating boundaries of the body, it is both empowering and threatening openness, which became particularly evident during the pandemic, when the encounter with the other body was potentially risky. In her text on affect and contamination, Agnieszka Anna Wołodźko ponders on this peculiar condition of the body, which she vividly calls porosity. As the dark history of the pandemic has shown, "our bodies have never been pure (…) we are porous and leaky bodies, conditioned by the encounters with multiple human and nonhuman bodies – be it other humans, animals, plants, bacteria viruses, yes viruses, particles, thoughts, experiences and minerals" (Wołodźko 2020: 214). From an evolutionary perspective, viruses have been part of the natural world for millions of years and have coexisted with humans throughout our shared biological history. The hostility of the COVID-19 virus is the crucial revision lesson that the purist image of the human body is nothing but a fragile construct of the mind, easily shattered in the face of nature's intentions.

While these insights may appear to be a digression from Foucault's concept of the body, I want to argue that the idea of the opacity, disjuncture, and fabrication of the body is encoded (sometimes latently, but more often – explicitly) in his work. For example, in "The Birth of the Clinic," he writes: "clinical experience sees a new space opening up before it: the tangible space of the body, which at the same time is that opaque mass in which secrets, invisible lesions, and the very mystery of origins lie hidden" (2003: 122). And further: the medicalization of the body has established the conceptual domain "in which the human body finds the concrete forms of its unity" (Ibid.: 129). Thus, the apparent unity and stable composition of the human body seem to be held together by strong discursive sutures whose nature is as artificial as the very notion of corporeal autonomy. Furthermore, as Rosalyn Diprose, who explores posthuman implications in Foucault's theorization of the body, argues, "Foucault's account of "*political* technologies of the body" proposes that human bodies are already technological (*techné*) by virtue of being enmeshed in the networks of power and circulating knowledges," and in this regard "politics targets the corporeal domain of the posthuman" (2009: 11). Paradoxically, disciplinary practices and the experience of the pandemic underscore the very same fact: that our human bodies are neither entirely human nor fully ours.

3 Human, Posthuman, More-than-Human Biopolitics

Elaborating and extending Foucault's notion of biopolitics, Giorgio Agamben argues that the ultimate operation lying at the core of the biopolitical machinery is the reduction of the human *bios* to zoē, *bare life* (1998: 12). In the context of the COVID-19 pandemic, however, this reduction was not imposed by governments, but rather by the virus itself, which represents a detour from classical human-centered theorizations of biopolitics and necessitates their reinterpretation. It may be superfluous, but it is still important to say that *life*, not human, is at the heart of biopolitics (*bios*, life).

Prior to moving on to more posthuman (more-than-human) accounts of Foucauldian biopolitics, it is important to remove latent humanist implications that are present in some of its interpretations. There is a general consensus among Foucault scholars that there is little consistency in his formulation of the concept of biopolitics, mainly because it was developed in parallel with his other major philosophical concepts, each of which determined the content of the concept of biopolitics at the time. For example, in the series "Security, Territory, Population," Foucault links the emergence of biopolitics to the biologization of the notion of humanity (*le genre humaine*), which is henceforth referred to as "a species of people" (*l'espèce humaine*) (Foucault 2009: 105). Such a shift of the focus from the political (humanity) to the *bio*political (species), however, does not indicate an increased anthropization of the political domain, but quite the opposite – its dehumanization, a break from sociocultural codes (discipline) to biological, zoological, natural codes. It is crucial to articulate that natural in the given context is not to be construed as physically or metaphysically correct, valid, or legitimate, as, semiotically speaking, a *primum signatum*, "the transcendental signified" (Derrida 1997: 20), but rather as an epistemological enigma; in fact, as Charles Darwin poignantly noted: "we shall at least be freed from the vain search for the undiscovered and undiscoverable essence of the term species" (qtd. from Clark 2020: 91). There is thus no essentialist fixed meaning of "a species of people" – and in this sense, as will be elaborated further, the Foucauldian notion of biopolitics has strong deconstructivist potential: it renounces the discovery of the political category of "people" and invents "people" through the intermediary of "a species of people" according to given criteria.

What are these criteria? To answer this question, another category needs to be introduced – that of populations. This term may be misleading because traditionally in political theory, "populations" have been associated with diverse groups of individuals within a society or political community and have depended heavily on anthropological notions of the state, citizenship, and governance. As a theorist of discourse and epistemes, Foucault cautions against a naïve understanding of "populations" as a construct of political theory and traces its emergence to the discourse of the natural sciences.[2] For him, popula-

2 For further elaboration on the relationship between biopolitical governmentality, naturalistic episteme, and populations, see: Petrina, D. 2017. "Daugiau nei apskaičiuojama, mažiau

tion is not a defined set of individuals and their characteristics, but rather a blend of the condition and object (object *because* it is a condition) of biopower; populations thus always require auxiliary categories, e.g., *working* population, *healthy* population, *fertile* population, and *ad infinitum* (Foucault 2009: 96–97). Eugene Thacker provides a succinct account of Foucault's concept of population. Following him, Thacker links this category to an epidemic of smallpox and thus to a new governmentality: while leprosy was based on the power to "exclude and divide bodies," the plague – on disciplinary observation, organization, and control, smallpox posed "the problem of multiplicities," which necessitated the new biopolitical apparatus that would "prevent the circulation of disease and still permit the circulation of people and goods" (Thacker 2011: 152). In this theoretical light, human populations are only one factor (albeit a very important one) among other factors – goods, disease, longevity, mortality, etc.; this factor is determined by quasi-natural events (Foucault 2009: 37), each of which (e.g. disaster, famine, decreased birth rate, or an epidemic like COVID-19) reconfigures and determines the content of what is considered a population – which thus requires a different approach to a *particular* population at a *particular* time in a *particular* space. To reiterate, populations as living multiplicities, as formulated by Thacker, are not a self-sufficient and self-explanatory phenomenon, but are a derivative of relations and connections with other social, political, cultural, economic, and most importantly, (quasi) natural phenomena.

This post-anthropocentric rereading of biopolitics (which, in fact, was never human-oriented, as the brief reconstruction of Foucault's arguments shows) highlights its conceptual link with new materialist scholarship, which is characterized by its preoccupation with a posthumanist agenda. In particular, Foucault's notion of "milieu" stands out as a theoretical arch connecting biopolitics with posthumanism. Foucault begins to work with the concept of "milieu" in his 1975–76 lecture series "Society Must Be Defended," where he provides a rather straightforward definition of the term that follows the mirror logic: he proposes to understand milieu as the effects of the environment on populations and vice versa – the effects of populations on their environments (2003: 245). The term becomes more nuanced in the following year's series of lectures, "Security, Territory, Population," where milieu is defined as a particular space in which "an indefinite series of multiple events" unfold, through which power apparatuses act on (intervene into) the environment and populations at a distance, in so doing altering the very materiality (Foucault 2009: 35–37). Fou-

nei vienas: populiacijos ir afekto santykis Michelio Foucault biopolitikos teorijoje." *Athena: filosofijos studijos*, No. 12, p. 196–211 (in Lithuanian).

cault would then continuously return to this concept, particularly emphasizing how the milieu produces its effects on the organism, drawing on Lamarck and Darwin's theories. The milieu, therefore, highlights the agential status of non-human (and even non-living) things; as Thomas Lemke rightfully notes, "agency is not exclusively a property of humans; rather, agential power originates in relations between humans and non-human entities. Also, the milieu articulates the link between the natural and the artificial without systematically distinguishing between them" (Lemke 2014: 8).

Viewed through this theoretical lens, the COVID-19 pandemic as the *milieu* offers several interesting practical-empirical insights into the posthuman implications of Foucauldian implicitly posthuman biopolitics *in actio*. First, as Mattias Lehtinen and Tuukka Brunila persuasively argue, the political ontological status of the pandemic was similar to that of war, "war against an invisible enemy" (Lehtinen, Brunila 2021: 2). The invisible enemy – the virus – required a novel political rationality, an inherently *bio*political rationality (or, perhaps, a more suitable term would be govern-*mentality*) – a life-centered one. While *practically* the course of action remained rather anthropocentric (it was *human* life that was saved), *epistemologically*, the category of human life proved to be not only insufficient but also even inadequate for understanding (and thus managing) the virus-induced pandemic. In essence, intervention in the milieu of the pandemic required a posthuman epistemology that interestingly combined such traditionally "human" disciplines as politics, sociology, and behavioral economics with medicine, biology, virology, environmental science, and similar ones. More than a testament to Foucault's observation of the medicalization of the state, it testifies to the changing nature of politics, whose subject is not human but rather transhuman, posthuman, or even nonhuman (as in the case of the virus[3]). Referring to the Butler's reinterpretation of the body that can never survive on its own, Lehtinen and Brunila problematize "the border between us and others, inherent to our institution of political

3 As argued extensively above, the management of the epidemics and biopolitics are the events of the same token, and in this respect biopolitics is a transhistorical phenomenon (which, in general, is in line with the Foucauldian (if rather incoherent) account of biopolitics). And yet, while the management of the previous epidemics (leprosy and plague) was also concerned with intervening in the causes of the infection, the measures taken (and thus the apparatuses employed) were largely human-centered. The management of the COVID-19 pandemic, being the product of a different *dispositif* (an assemblage of material-discursive conditions of the phenomenon), was founded on different epistemological premises (a different "field of knowledge" *qua* the possibility of knowledge) and therefore the majority of the tools used (e.g., the knowledge corpus of molecular biology, statistical representation, and data-driven forecasting and regulation, to name a few) could be considered posthuman.

ontology." The reconfiguration of our political ontology, brought about by the pandemic, underscores "the flickering character of drawing such borders, and even for its impossibility." (Ibid.: 14). The agential status of the virus (virus as the hyperobject, as Timothy Morton would call it (2013) (and the high possibility of the pandemic recurring in the future) is living proof of the obsolescence of anthropocentric biopolitics.

Second, as I have argued in the preceding section, the intervention in the pandemic milieu targeted the incompleteness and imperfection of the human body and its meta/physical vulnerability. A collective of authors – Anne Wagner, Aleksandra Matulewska, and Sarah Marusek – have emphasized the reappearance of the disciplinary paradigm within the horizon of biopolitics. In their account of the management of the pandemic (the research was ongoing throughout the entire pandemic), the authors mention such disciplinary techniques as restrictions on mobility and transportation, exploitation of the medical workforce, quarantine, spatial, and behavioral regulations (e.g., social distancing and wearing masks), and physical and digital surveillance – in short, measures ideally suited to the quest to prevent the circulation of disease and preserve the circulation of people and goods, as Thacker described it. According to them, this has led to the formation of a new distribution of power, which they call *Pandemica Panoptica*, that "subjugates individual bodies, and enforces proper ways of body movement or retreat, as dictated by the appropriate regulating authorities within determined spatial and temporal framework(s)" (Wagner et al. 2022: 1084).

While the management of the pandemic relied heavily on "good old-fashioned" discipline, it does not present a complete picture: in fact, and even more so, the management of the pandemic can be characterized by what Deleuze called "free-floating control," which operates by transforming individuals into "dividuals" (Deleuze 1992: 4–5). Numerous authors (I will mention only a few in a cursory manner) have highlighted the strong reliance of COVID-19 governance on the repertoire of techniques developed and applied in "control societies." Kelum Jayasinghe et al. emphasize the intersection between biopolitics and calculative technologies (2022), Deborah Lupton raises the problems of digital surveillance and control accompanied by algorithmic injustices during the COVID-19 crisis (2022), while Handan Vicdan describes the process of the platformization of COVID-19 that gave rise to what he calls biosocial surveillance (2020). The overarching affective motif of these works is an alarming suspicion of the computational nature of biopower – in the context of the pandemic, the mechanisms of data collection, use, and storage, and more generally, the not-yet-fully-understood and not-yet-fully-understandable transformation of entire populations into data, individuals into dividuals.

This observation resonates with Lemke's interpretation of another less popular Foucault's idea, that of "the government of things" that replaces "the government of souls and bodies" (Lemke 2014: 8). Such a government, as Lemke comprehensively explains, "works on empirical quantities: on geophysical phenomena (climate, water supply, geographical data, etc.) as well as on bio-demographic facts (birth and death rates, health status, life span, the production of wealth, etc.). By statistically aggregating men on the level of populations, they finally become calculable and measurable and could be conceived of as physical phenomena themselves" (Ibid.). People are no longer people, not even populations or "a species of people" – they are now data and datasets. The pandemic has set the stage for the reinforcement of digital or data-driven biopolitics, which exemplifies the *negative* posthuman scenario that should be countered with *positive* posthuman alternatives.

Ultimately, as outlined in previous arguments, the agency of the virus and datafication testify to the conceptual, theoretical, and methodological incompleteness of the notion of the human in the realm of biopolitics in general and post-pandemic biopolitics in particular. In fact, Donna Haraway made this argument more than 20 years ago, stating that "Michael (*sic!*) Foucault's biopolitics is a flaccid premonition of cyborg politics, a very open field" (1991: 150). Foucault's concept of milieu is based on the fact that humans form assemblages with many others – other humans, animals, plants, places, whole natural and non-natural environments, including radical others – such as the inorganic virus and techno-material digital infrastructures, as in the COVID-19 pandemic. This "open field," as Haraway called it, requires the metaphorical "death of man" to make room for conceptual tools that are capable of bearing the weight of the surplus of meanings that are otherwise suspended and unregistered by the category of "human" – *posthuman* (dislocation of boundaries between human and non-human entities), *transhuman* (transcending the limits of human subjects), *non-human* (radically different epistemologies and phenomenologies), *more-than-human* (entire assemblages, infra/structures, and ecosystems), etc. In a similar vein, van Wichelen claims that Foucauldian biopolitics has always been a "more-than-human biopolitics" because of "his (*Foucault's*) conceptual equipment (*dispositif*, governmentality, and millieu) and his privileging of genealogies and practices as non-linear and entangled with "things" (van Wichelen 2020: 171). This brings us to our final object of inquiry, the genealogy of the post-pandemic subject.

4 Techniques of the Self beyond the Self: On Post-pandemic Health Politics

On March 28, 1984, Foucault delivered his last lecture – he decided to dedicate his final series of lectures to the problem of courage and truth. His final words were:

> Only by deciphering the truth of self in this world, deciphering oneself with mistrust of oneself and the world [...] will enable us to have access to the true life.
>
> 2011: 338

At first, these words sound rather "humanistic," if not dull. They sound quite different; however, if we recall a painful yet important fact of Foucault's biography, he was already suffering from AIDS complications by then. The same year Foucault uttered these words, he succumbed to HIV and died. At that time, the AIDS epidemic was raging, claiming most of the lives of the homosexual men population. The acceptance of Foucault's last invitation to seek "access to the true life" is not only a reflection on strikingly timely wise words in the early post-pandemic period (as they were inspired by Foucault's own uneven battle with the virus) but also a tribute to the philosopher paid by the reactivating his thought with renewed vigor when it is desperately needed.

I will, therefore, pay this tribute by contributing to the collective writing of the post-pandemic "story without the subject" (Herbrechter 2013: 12) – at least the subject as we know it. Foucault's conceptual framework of the "genealogy of the subject" is essentially the methodological exemplification of the "mistrust of oneself and the world," of which he speaks in his last lecture, since its fundamental proposition is that the subject is not a metaphysical entity, but a historical construct. In the context of posthumanism, as Stefan Herbrechter persuasively argues, genealogy "exposes the 'cardinal sins' of 'Western metaphysics': logocentrism, phallocentrism and anthropocentrism" and "problematizes a monolithic view of humanism by locating a radical self-criticism already within the humanist tradition and on this basis, by arguing for a non-normative, 'post-foundational' humanism '*that refuses to define the human*' and thus escapes the '*tyranny of naming and quantifying the human*'" (Ibid.: 77; Hallliwel and Mousley 2003: 9–10). What would then this critical genealogy of the post-pandemic subject, based on "mistrust of oneself," look like – at least fragmentarily represented?

An important dimension of the genealogy of the subject is Foucault's concept of "technologies of the self." This concept encompasses technologies, practices, and discourses that the individual uses to construct "the hermeneutics of the self" (Foucault 1988: 17) that would function as a counternarrative to hegemonic social, political, and even philosophical and scientific epistemologies – which, as a result, would allow access to true life, as Foucault worded it. Foucault himself stresses the need for a balance between the subject and the world to live "the true life," which, in Haraway's words, creates an "open field" of politics. Inventing oneself as a subject is an essentially political act, particularly when one's subjectivity goes against the very *rules* of subjectivity – autonomy, self-sufficiency, and self-regulation. If we understand anything about the pandemic, it is that this auto-/self-component is the problematic part: not only are we vulnerable and weak in the face of a destructive virus, but even in calm times, we are never "on our own" and are always interdependent with others. The confinements, quarantines, and spatial regulations evoked a sense of claustrophobia that eerily translates into an onto-epistemic situation of the subject trapped within itself, as if in an echo chamber.

This claustrophobic feeling (*of* oneself being *with* oneself *for* oneself) has proven once again that the ground of subjectivity is shaky and unstable. Paradoxically, what gives it a more solid foundation is not a paranoid adherence to the limits of one's own human body but an acknowledgment of the inescapable openness to others – both human and nonhuman, reliance and dependence on them – that paves the way for posthuman technologies of the self. As Elaine Graham points out, "posthuman technologies of the self are articulated in such new locations as cyberspace, laboratories or in the neuroclinic or the sperm bank" (2004: 21). Posthuman technologies of the self must therefore take into account our existential indeterminacy and incompleteness, which is characterized by precarity and vulnerability on the one hand, but also by creativity and experimental potential of joining new assemblages and learning to be in them on the other. Since vulnerability is a part of the equation, posthuman technologies of the self should be structured around the epistemological-affective core of care – care for oneself, other humans, non-humans, the planet, and all its parts. Care is crucial for what Francesca Ferrando calls "radical healing," which may involve "staying with the trouble" (Haraway 2016) – the trouble from which the world has yet to recover – which is only possible if we embark on "a transformative, restorative, and radically healing journey: ethical, to the ontological core" (Ferrando 2020: 157).

The idea of radical healing and ontological restoration, especially in the post-pandemic context, requires me to address the subject of health. Health, understood in a neoliberal episteme in categories of privacy and individual capacity, and in this sense – as a property – should be redefined not only to free it from its normative character but also to make it more inclusive of many others who participate in the co-constitution of our health. In her recent book, "The Virus Touch: Theorizing Epidemic Media," Bishnupriya Ghosh presents a strikingly apt reconfiguration of health as a "multispecies politics." She writes: "Health is at once a complex multiform *horizon* for multispecies cohabitation and a concrete public good toward which we strive. In other words, health structures the ethical call to symbiotic agreements as a *situated place-based* politics. With each epidemic, we learn more about what is to be done about health" (Ghosh 2023: 73). The painful yet very valuable lesson of COVID-19 is that the health of the population, "a species of people," as the ultimate biopolitical goal, will never cease to fail as long as it remains constrained by human-centered epistemes; posthuman biopolitics thus shifts its focus from individual health as *a goal* to collective health as *a horizon* through continuous and never-ending radical planetary healing.

Foucault's favorite philosopher, from whom he borrowed the method of genealogy, Friedrich Nietzsche's famous proclamation in 1882 that "God is dead" was considered scandalous and utterly unbelievable at the time; nonetheless, it became a philosophical motto of the post-metaphysical philosophical tradition for centuries. Foucault's words about "the death of man" could be prophetic in two ways: either literally – as the death of humanity brought about by impeding ecological disaster, man-made causes, or another epidemic, this time more violent and deadly in its nature, or hopefully, as the long overdue end of the genealogy of the *human* subject, to be then replaced by the genealogy of the *posthuman* – which, startling as it may sound, has already begun.

References

Agamben, Giorgio. 1998. *Homo Sacer: Sovereign Power and Bare Life*, translated by Daniel Heller-Roazen. Stanford University Press.

Anderson, Ian. 1995. "Bodies, Disease and the Problem of Foucault". *Social Analysis: The International Journal of Social and Cultural Practice*, No. 37, p. 67–81.

Bratton, Benjamin. 2021. *The Revenge of the Real: Politics for a Post-pandemic World*. London, New York: Verso.

Canguilhem, Georges. *The Normal and the Pathological*. Translated by Carolyn Fawcett. Zone Books, 1991.

Clark, Bruce. 2020. "Machines, Ai, Cyborgs, Systems", edited by Sherryl Vint. *After the Human: Culture, Theory, and Criticism in the 21st Century*. Cambridge: Cambridge University Press, p. 91–104.

"Coronavirus and Philosophers" [online]. 2020. *European Journal of Psychoanalysis*. February 2020 – May 2020, https://www.journal-psychoanalysis.eu/articles/coronavirus-and-philosophers/. Accessed 26 December 2023.

Deleuze, Gilles. 1992. "Postscript on the Societies of Control", *October*, Vol. 59 (Winter 1992), p. 3–7.

Deleuze, Gilles, Guattari, Félix. 2000. *Anti-Oedipus: Capitalism and Schizophrenia*, translated by Hurley Robert, Seem Mark, and Lane Helen. Minneapolis: University of Minnesota Press.

Derrida, Jacques. 1997. *Of Grammatology*, translated by Spivak Gayatri Chakravorty. Baltimore and London: The John Hopkins University Press.

Diprose, Rosalyn. 2009. "Toward an ethico-politics of the posthuman: Foucault and Merleau-Ponty". *Parrhesia*, No. 8, p. 7–19.

Ferrando, Francesca. 2020. "Posthuman Feminist Ethics: Unveiling Ontological Radical Healing". Edited by Thomsen, Mads Rosendahl, Wamberg, Jacob. *The Bloomsbury Handbook of Posthumanism*. London: Bloomsbury, p. 141–160.

Foucault, Michel. 1970. *The Order of Things: An Archaeology of the Human Sciences*, translated by A. Sheridan. New York: Vintage Books.

Foucault, Michel. 1976. *The Birth of the Clinic: An Archaeology of Medical Perception*, translated by A. Sheridan. London: Routledge.

Foucault, Michel. 1988. "Technologies of the Self", edited by Luther Martin, Huck Gutman, and Patrick Hutton. *Technologies of the Self: A Seminar with Michel Foucault*. Massachusetts: The University of Massachusetts Press.

Foucault, Michel. 1995. *Discipline and Punish: The Birth of the Prison*, translated by A. Sheridan. New York: Vintage Books.

Foucault, Michel. 2003. *Society Must be Defended: Lectures at the College de France 1975–1976*, translated by. D. Macey. New York: Picador.

Foucault, Michel. 2004. *The Birth of Biopolitics, Lectures at the College de France 1978–1979*, translated by G. Burchell. New York: Palgrave.

Foucault, Michel. 2009. *Security, Territory, Population: Lectures at the College de France 1977–1978*, translated by G. Burchell. New York: Palgrave Macmillan.

Foucault, Michel. 2011. *The Courage of Truth*, edited by Gros Frédéric, Davidson, Arnold. Translated by Graham Burchell. Basingstoke: Palgrave Macmillan.

Ghosh, Bishnupriya. 2023. *The Virus Touch: Theorizing Epidemic Media*. Durham: Duke University Press.

Graham, Elaine. 2004. "Post/Human Conditions", *Theology & Sexuality*, Vol. 10, No. 2, p. 10–32.

Halliwelll, Martin, Mousley, Andy. 2003. *Critical Humanisms: Humanist/Anti-Humanist Dialogues*. Edinburgh: Edinburgh University Press.

Haraway, Donna. 1991. *Simians, Cyborgs, and Women: The Reinvention of Nature*. New York: Routledge.

Haraway, Donna. 2016. *Staying with the Trouble: Making Kin in the Chthulucene*. Durham: Duke University Press.

Hayles, Katherine. 2021. "Novel Corona: Posthuman Virus". *Critical Inquiry*, Vol. 47 (Winter 2021), p. 68–72.

Herbrechter, Stefan. 2013. *Posthumanism: A Critical Analysis*. London & New York: Bloomsbury Publishing.

Jayasinghe, Kelum, Jayasinghe, Tarosha, Wijethilake, Chaminda, and Adhikari, Pawan. 2022. "Bio-Politics and Calculative Technologies in COVID-19 Governance: Reflections from England". *International Journal of Health Policy and Management*, vol. 11, no. 10, p. 2189–2197.

Jonutytė, Jurga. 2022. "An "Experiment" of Anti-Ableistic Equality During the COVID-19 Pandemic". *Athena: filosofijos studijos*, No. 17, p. 173–187.

Lehtinen, Mattias, and Brunila, Tuukka. 2021. "Political Ontology of the Pandemic: Sovereign Power and the Management of Affects through the Political Ontology of War". *Hypothesis and Theory*, Vol. 3, p. 1–17.

Lemke, Thomas. 2014. "New Materialisms: Foucault and the 'Government of Things'". *Theory, Culture & Society*, Vol. 34, No. 4, p. 1–23.

Lupton, Deborah. 2022. "The quantified pandemic: Digitised Surveillance, Containment and Care in Response to the Covid-19 Crisis", edited by Sarah Pink, Martin Berg, Deborah Lupton, and Minna Ruckenstein. *Everyday Automation: Experiencing and Anticipating Emerging Technologies*. London and New York: Routledge, p. 59–72.

Markula, Pirkko. 2006. "Deleuze and the body without organs: Disreading the fit feminine identity". *Journal of Sport and Social Issues*. Vol. 30, No. 1, p. 29–44.

Morton, Timothy. 2013. *Hyperobjects: Philosophy and Ecology after the End of the World*. Minnesota: University of Minnesota Press.

Newman, Saul, Topuzovski Tihomir (eds.). 2021. *The Posthuman Pandemic*. London and New York: Bloomsbury Publishing.

Petrina, Denis. 2017. "Daugiau nei apskaičiuojama, mažiau nei vienas: populiacijos ir afekto santykis Michelio Foucault biopolitikos teorijoje". *Athena: filosofijos studijos*, No. 12, p. 196–211.

Protevi, John. 2015. "Body", edited by Lawlor, Leonard, and Nale, John. *The Cambridge Foucault Lexicon*. Cambridge: Cambridge University Press, p. 51–56.

Rose, Nikolas. 2007. *The Politics of Life Itself: Biomedicine, Power, and Subjectivity in the Twenty-First Century*. Princeton: Princeton University Press.

Shildrick, Margrit. 2009. *Dangerous Discourses of Disability, Subjectivity and Sexuality*. New York: Palgrave Macmillan.

Thacker, Eugene. 2011. "Necrologies; or the Death of the Body Politics", edited by Patricia Ticineto Clough, Craig Willse. *Beyond Biopolitics: Essays on the Governance of Life and Death*. Durham: Duke University Press, p. 139–162.

Van Wichelen, Sonja. 2020. "More-than-Human Biopolitics". Edited by Sherryl Vint. *After the Human: Culture, Theory, and Criticism in the 21st Century*. Cambridge: Cambridge University Press, p. 161–176.

Vicdan, Handan. 2020. "Platformization of COVID and the Rise of Biosocial Surveillance". *Markets, Globalization and Development Review*, Vol. 5, no. 3, p. 1–9.

Wagner, Anne, Matulewska, Aleksandra, and Marusek, Sarah. 2022. "*Pandemica Panoptica*: Biopolitical Management of Viral Spread in the Age of Covid-19". *International Journal for the Semiotics of Law*, Vol. 35, p. 1081–1117.

Wołodźko, Agnieszka. 2020. "Living within affect as contamination: breathing in between numbers", *Capacious: Journal for Emerging Affect Inquiry*, Vol. 2, No. 1–2, p. 212–224.

CHAPTER 6

Transindividual Biopolitics

Audronė Žukauskaitė

Abstract

The recent attempts to interpret the COVID-19 pandemic in terms of biopolitics, such as the one provided by Giorgio Agamben, prove that the notion of biopolitics should be radically reconsidered. Biopolitics should be understood not in terms of sovereign power but as a form of interaction between natural potentials, individuals, and technical objects. For this reason, I would like to introduce Gilbert Simondon's notion of the transindividual, consider its recent interpretations by Étienne Balibar and Bernard Stiegler, and outline a project of transindividual biopolitics. The COVID-19 pandemic and the attempt to create a collective immunity (or "herd immunity") can be seen as a transindividual condition, where every individual is confronted with something pre-individual (namely, a virus) and, at the same time, with other individuals with whom it shares its immunity, thus creating a relationship of responsibility and solidarity. This example of transindividual can be reconsidered as a new mode of biopolitics: biopolitics is conceptualized not as a negative force but as an affirmative interaction between human and nonhuman forces. Such reconceptualization of biopolitics would change the focus from the opposition between a malicious sovereign and subjugated individuals to the affirmative model of transindividual communities. It means that the anthropocentric model of biopolitics should embrace both the biological and geo-bio-chemical conditions of the planet and the geological timescale of deep time.

Keywords

the pre-individual – individual – transindividual – biopolitics – cosmopolitics

As the difficult time of the pandemic passes by, many authors struggle to define what happened to us and our society. What new forms of political and ethical engagement can we obtain from the experience of the COVID-19 pandemic? Can we see this experience as a threshold that opens new forms of community? What this experience makes clear is that the relationship between an individual and society should be reconsidered because the

 | DOI:10.1163/9789004748187_008

pandemic experience gives clear evidence that we live in a posthuman condition: the human individual is invaded and contaminated by nonhuman viruses and can survive only by relying on new technologies of vaccination. The emergence of new zoonotic viruses can be seen as an effect of human manipulation of nonhuman animals. In this sense, the human individual is trapped in a strange combination of technology and animality. As Rosi Braidotti points out, "This combination of ambivalent elements in relation to the Fourth Industrial Revolution and the Sixth Extinction is the trademark of the posthuman condition" (Braidotti 2020). This posthuman post-pandemic condition needs a new conceptualization and a new conceptual vocabulary. Now more than ever it is clear that we cannot rely on the classical distinctions between individual and society, nature and culture, and culture and technology. In this respect the notion of biopolitics, as it was formulated by Michel Foucault and Giorgio Agamben, also needs to be reconceptualized. Conventional biopolitics is structured around the figure of the sovereign and its power to exercise control over individual bodies or populations. However, we should ask if this approach is still relevant and appropriate.

In his latest book, *Where Are We Now? The Epidemic as Politics* (2021), Agamben demonstrates the failure to analyse the pandemic situation in terms of sovereignty. As you know, Agamben interprets the recent health crisis as a state of exception and compares the restrictions issued by local governments with Hitler's declaration of the state of exception in 1933 and the abolition of the Weimar Constitution. Agamben's argument that the pandemic is a secret plan created by governments to implement some special measures that would turn us, human individuals, into mere biological creatures puts into doubt his entire project of biopolitics. This leads to the idea that the opposition between sovereign power (or the government or the state) and the allegedly oppressed individual is misleading and that a negative model of biopolitics should be replaced by a more positive one. Biopolitics should be understood not in terms of sovereign power but as a form of interaction between various individuals, technical objects, and natural forces attempting to solve particular problems. For this reason, I would like to introduce Gilbert Simondon's notion of the transindividual, consider its recent interpretations by Étienne Balibar and Bernard Stiegler, and outline a project of transindividual biopolitics.

1 Simondon's Notion of the Transindividual

Gilbert Simondon created a theory of individuation, or ontogenesis, according to which individuals are only temporal phases of permanent becoming. In

Individuation in Light of Notions of Form and Information (2020), Simondon compares physical, biological, psychical, and technical individuation. In contrast to physical individuation, which is completed when certain conditions are exhausted, biological and psychical individuation is in continuous transformation through interaction both with the pre-individual and its milieu. Not only physical and biological individuals develop, evolve, and change; human individuals can also be conceived as a system of three successive phases of being: "the pre-individual phase, the individuated phase, and the transindividual phase, all of which [...] correspond to what is designated by the concepts of nature, individual, and spirituality. The subject is [...] the condensed and systematized unity of the three phases of being" (Simondon 2020: 348–9). This makes us think that the human subject is constituted somewhere in between the pre-individual phase (which stands for nature) and "spirituality" (which stands for culture and technology). Let's take a closer look at this definition.

Simondon takes the notion of the pre-individual phase from physics, namely, from the thermodynamic notion of metastable equilibrium. A stable equilibrium is achieved when all potential energies are actualized and all transformations achieved; by contrast, a metastable equilibrium is a system that is neither stable nor unstable but is charged with potentials for becoming and contains enough potential to "produce an abrupt alteration leading to a new, equally metastable structuration" (Simondon 2020: 369). As one of many examples of metastable equilibrium, Simondon discusses the duality of a photon, which can be regarded both as a particle and a wave and both as a physical individual and as a certain amount of energy, which is capable of potential change. Thus, a metastable equilibrium, which defines the pre-individual state, can be considered a reservoir of potential energy, which is the condition for transformation and change, engendering the process of individuation. Simondon often refers to the pre-individual in pre-Socratic terms; in other words, for him, nature is *apeiron*, that is, a real pre-individual potential, which makes individuation possible.

Thus, the pre-individual potential initiates the process of individuation; however, what this process creates is neither an individual (as an atom) nor a society (as a whole) but the transindividual phase. The notion of the transindividual not only replaces the dualism between an individual and a society but also deconstructs both terms by revealing that both of them consist of multiple relationships. Every individual is connected with pre-individual potential (which also can be described as a milieu) and with other individuals. In this sense, an individual is never completed and bounded onto itself but is extended into both sides – to the side of the pre-individual, which is full of potential and indeterminacy, and to the side of the transindividual, which is transpersonal and collective. However, this collective state is understood not as an agglomerate of individuals but as a collective being, which is traversed by pre-individual indeterminacy. As Simondon points out, "it is precisely based on this position of the unresolved in man, within this not-yet-individuated charge of reality, that man seeks out his fellow man to form a group in which he will find presence through a second individuation. [...] the individual has conserved the pre-individual with it, and all individuals together thus have a sort of unstructured ground based upon which a new individuation can occur" (Simondon 2020: 340). This means that every individual is prolonged beyond itself and forms relationships with the real world and vice versa: every collective is made of relationships, which are constituted not between formed individuals but between processes of individuation.

In this respect, Simondon distinguishes between an interindividual and transindividual relation: the interindividual relation is established between completed and self-sufficient individuals, whereas the transindividual relation passes through every individual in such a way that they form a system that "contains potentials and metastability, expectation and tension" (Simondon 2020: 339). This means that the transindividual phase can be described as a bundle of multiple relations both with the pre-individual potential and with other individuals who share this pre-individual charge. It is this unresolved potential that makes further individuation possible, creating "tension and potentials for becoming-other, for recommencing an individuation that is not destructive of the first" (Simondon 2020: 340). It seems that for Simondon, the notion of the transindividual refers to a realm beyond the limits of the individual, which opens new individuations. However, we should ask what Simondon means by this pre-individual charge and what kind of potential these individuals are sharing.

Another definition of the transindividual appears in Simondon's book *On the Mode of Existence of Technical Objects* (2017), where the transindividual phase is related to the invention of a technical object. Simondon argues that the relation between an inventor (a subject) and a technical object creates a special mode of relationship which he calls transindividual: "the technical object insofar as it has been invented, thought and willed, and taken up [*assumé*] by a human subject, becomes the medium [*le support*] and symbol of this relationship, which we would like to name *transindividual*" (Simondon 2017: 252). Technical invention creates a special trans-human relation where individuals are connected by the pre-individual potential. "An inter-human relation that is the model of *transindividuality* is thus created through the intermediary of the technical object. This can be understood as a relationship that does not relate individuals by means of their constituted individuality separating them from one another, nor by means of what is identical in every human subject, for instance, the *a priori* forms of sensibility, but by means of this weight [*charge*] of pre-individual reality, this weight of nature that is preserved with the individual being, and which contains potentials and virtualities" (Simondon 2017: 253). It is important to point out that for Simondon, a technical object is not something artificial but, on the contrary, something that appears as a prolongation or an extension of nature. A good example here is the invention of the Guimbal turbine: it is a turbine that uses the river as a driving force; however, the more effective it is, the more heat it creates, and finally, the engine might burn out. At this point, it needs some concretization or some technical invention to solve the problem of overheating. It is the inventor who makes the technical system evolve by adding an invention that allows the turbine to cool down: the current of the river forces the turbine to move and, at the same time, cools it down and prevents it from overheating. This invention not only resolves technical problems but also connects a natural milieu (the river), the inventor, and a technical object by recurrent causality.

That means that through the knowledge of technical objects, an individual (an inventor) is related both to nature and its potentiality and to other individuals. The transindividual phase means the exteriorization of an individual, its folding out, and, at the same time, its relationship with other individuals, created through technical imagination and inventiveness. As Muriel Combes points out, "the invented technical object becomes the bearer of information for other subjects, which, through the intermediary of the object, then assembles their inventive and organizational capacities with those of the inventor" (Combes 2013: 77). At the same time Simondon points out that technical activity is not the only mode which helps to create a collective and that it is only in certain cases that a collective is born out of technical activity.

This quite enigmatic notion of the transindividual was interpreted by Étienne Balibar and Bernard Stiegler, who expanded the notion of the transindividual to the sphere of collective imagination and technicity in general. But before examining their interpretations, we should take into account that other interpreters, such as Muriel Combes, define the transindividual in terms of the real: "Thus these shares of nature, of real potential, are what link individuals to one another in the collective; it is because of them that constituted individuals can enter into relation with one another and constitute a collective; these shares are potentials actually existing *as potentials* even though they are not actually structured, they are what is not individuated in individuals" (Combes 2013: 47). Combes points out that the transindividual collective is of a physical nature – "in the sense in which pre-Socratic thinkers are said to be physicians, thinkers of nature, thinkers of the *physis*" (Combes 2013: 48). Simondon distinguishes between the subjective and objective transindividual: subjective transindividual refers to subjective affect when the individual discovers its more-than-individuality, some external reality that is both pre-individual and common to other individuals; the objective transindividual refers to an operation through which these common shares are collectively structured (Combes 2013: 48). In this respect, Simondon situates the transindividual within physical reality taking place in the real. As Combes points out, "Such a gesture avoids any formalist conception of the constitution of the collective by contract, and even any thinking in terms of sovereignty, whose sole concern is to guarantee the legitimacy of the subsumption of society within the State. Consequently, in his inquiry into the real constitution of the collective, Simondon [...] situates himself in a line of inquiry striving to think the political *outside* the horizon of the legitimization of sovereignty" (Combes 2013: 48). Thus, as I suggested earlier, the transindividual could be interpreted as a (bio)political theory grounded not on the notion of sovereignty but on the idea of commonality.

2 Balibar's Notion of the Transindividual

The notion of the transindividual was recently discussed in Étienne Balibar's book *Spinoza, The Transindividual* (2020). Balibar supports Simondon's idea of individuation and argues that the ontology of individuals should be replaced by the ontology of relations. This ontology of relations is oriented towards individual becoming, collective transformation, and plasticity of institutions, and in this sense, it overcomes the opposition between necessity and freedom (Balibar 2020: 138). It is because of these characteristics, which transgress the established philosophical order, that Balibar is interested in Simondon. He uses Simondon's notion of the transindividual to re-interpret Spinoza, Marx, and Freud, even though the term is applied a posteriori because it was not available when these authors were writing their works. Balibar interprets these three philosophical examples as the modes of relational ontology where individuals affect each other and exchange their parts (Spinoza), are related to each other through commodity fetishism (Marx), or through the relations of identification and desire that are structured around the Other (Freud). Let's take a closer look at these examples of the transindividual.

The first example of the transindividual Balibar extracts from Spinoza even though Simondon denies any debt to Spinoza, whom he sees as a "pantheistic" philosopher negating individuality as such (Balibar 2020: 45). Spinoza explains that an individual cannot persist without exchanging some parts with other individuals that form its environment. Every individual constantly abandons some of their parts and incorporates parts of other individuals. As Balibar points out, "to be able to exchange parts with others, each individual must undergo a *virtual decomposition* [...]. Individuals mutually modify each other or 'mingle' with one another because they exchange constituent parts [...] decomposing into more basic parts and recomposed into relatively autonomous units" (Balibar 2020: 54–55). Relying on this, Balibar argues that Spinozian ontology is primarily based on individuations (exchange and variation of individual forms) and individualizations (the powers and capacities that an individual possesses) rather than individuals. Every individual is a transindividual to the extent that individuals are decomposing and recomposing themselves, constantly exchanging their "parts" and "affections" between themselves. In this respect, the Spinozian ontology reminds me of Margulis' notion of symbiosis and her idea that all life forms are the result of incessant symbiotic relations. The idea of the virtual decomposition of bodies is also useful in thinking about the pandemic condition where viruses are exchanged between bodies in such a way that increases or decreases their capacity for living.

Another two examples of the transindividual come from a different context: these are the Marxist notion of commodity fetishism and the Freudian notion of desire. According to Marx, in the case of commodity fetishism, we see a relation of double alienation – alienation as a relation to things that appear as commodities and alienation as a relationship with other individuals that appear as participants in the production process: workers, owners, merchants, etc. Balibar thinks that this double alienation can be seen as an interesting example of the transindividual: private individuals relate between themselves not directly binding to each other but through their relationship to commodity exchange – individuals relate through the relationships between objects. "Thus it is the system of things exchanged against each other, objectified in monetary expression and more generally that of an *object-value*, 'sensible suprasensible', which not only *makes* individuals *see* the 'society' of which they are members, but also *establishes* it, since without this representation [...] individual producers *would not exist for one another*, nor would they form 'society'" (Balibar 2020: 150). Balibar sees this alienation not as something that destroys transindividuality but rather constitutes it.

Another example of the transindividual Balibar discovers in Freudian psychoanalysis, where "the moment of the transindividual" appears in the tension between the individual and the collective desire. Both individual and collective desire imply either an identification with an object or an identification with another subject, which grants the reality of this object. Balibar refers to an intrinsic duality of the identificatory model: "on the one hand [...] there is what Freud calls *the overvaluation of the object* (or the denial of its defects); on the other [...] *the suspension of the judgment of reality*, or, better, the 'delegation' to the other of *the testing of reality*, which the subject renounces for himself in installing truth in the other (who can be a leader, a teacher, even a professor or an ideology)" (Balibar 2020: 168). In this respect, desire represents a double relation, first to the object of desire and then to the other individual, which legitimates this object as desirable. Referring to Marx and Freud, Balibar argues that the construction of the transindividual has a quasi-transcendental function in the sense that it both *institutes* the individual and the collective and simultaneously *denatures* them (Balibar 2020: 183). However, I would argue that it is precisely this quasi-transcendental function that makes Balibar's interpretation problematic.

What gets lost in this interpretation is the relation with pre-individual potential, which is the necessary condition for individuation to occur and which, for Simondon, comes from material reality or "nature." However, commodity fetishism, as described by Marx, or the processes of identification and desire, as described by Freud, represent interindividual rather than transindividual relationships. The case of Spinoza is much more complicated because, in Spinoza, the subject is not cleanly differentiated from nature and can be considered as a part of it. As was said earlier, Simondon denied any debt to Spinoza, whom he saw as a "pantheistic" philosopher, negating individuality as such; regardless of this, Balibar's reading of Spinoza as a philosophy of the transindividual is more convincing than his reading of Freud or Marx. In Spinoza, the individual is trying to carve out its form from nature, and therefore, it has support in ontological reality, whereas in Freud and Marx, the individual is related to the collective via a purely imaginary – or quasi-transcendental – form of relations. In this respect, we are dealing with interindividual rather than transindividual relationships.

3 Stiegler on the Transindividual

Another attempt to interpret the notion of the transindividual belongs to Bernard Stiegler. As Jason Read points out, "Stiegler's reading of Simondon returns to the initial identification of transindividuality and technology; transindividuality is the technical milieu, and this milieu, in the form of artefacts and writings, forms the basis of collective history and individual memory" (Read 2017: 170). For Stiegler, technology represents a specific moment when human interiority is exteriorized and extended through the use of technological objects. "The movement inherent in this process of exteriorization is paradoxical: Leroi-Gourhan in fact says that it is the tool, that is, *tekhnē*, that invents the human, not the human who invents the technical. Or again: the human invents himself in the technical by inventing the tool – by becoming exteriorized techno-logically" (Stiegler 1998: 141). In this respect, technology not only has a specific spatial dimension – it forces a human individual to turn himself or herself out into exteriority – but also a temporal dimension: the technological object becomes a place for memory and history. Stiegler refers to Husserl's analysis of internal time consciousness, which is divided between actual perception (primary retention and primary protention) and our imagination (secondary retention and secondary protention). In addition to this schema, Stiegler suggests what he names tertiary retention – retention, which is inscribed in memory of technical objects. It is an artificial or technological memory, such as writing or recording, which compresses actual primary and imaginary secondary retentions. This technological memory can be externalized and detached from an actual individual and shared by other individuals and even other generations. Stiegler argues that this technological memory is transindividual in the Simondonian sense.

Stiegler differentiates between three types of memory: the genetic memory of the biological individual, the epigenetic memory of the existential individual, and the epiphylogenetic (technological) memory, which is transindividual and which designates technicity in general (Stiegler 1998: 177). For Stiegler, genetic memory follows a "program" in a quasi-deterministic biological sense, whereas epigenesis is the development of a unique individual, which, unfortunately, is finite and disappears when its life ends. It is only with epiphylogenesis, in other words, with technological artificial memory, that epigenesis can be retained and memorized: "this epigenetic sedimentation, a memorization of what has come to pass, is what is called the past, what we shall name the *epiphylogenesis* of man, meaning the conservation, accumulation, and sedimentation of successive epigeneses, mutually articulated. Epiphylogenesis is a break with pure life…" (Stiegler 1998: 140). Epiphylogenesis, or tertiary retention, allows one to access the past that one never lived in and share it with other individuals and other generations.

Technological memory, or tertiary retention, is a transindividual condition that is necessary for organizing the collective. Psychic and collective individuation is always co-evolving together with technical individuation. In this respect, Stiegler follows Simondon's notion of the transindividual. And yet, in contrast to Simondon, Stiegler argues that tertiary retention, or technological memory, could lead both to transindividuation and disindividuation. In the case of transindividuation, an individual is confronted with the history of technological invention and transformation; therefore, its individuation is intensified and may create new social and political forms of solidarity. As Read points out, "It is through this history of transindividuality, a history of its changing technological and social transformation of this process of inscription, this grammatization, that Stiegler approaches political economy. [...] For Stiegler, this grammatization somewhat anachronistically makes possible the figure of the citizen" (Read 2016: 174). Transindividual inscription carries within itself not only the history of technology but also the history of social institutions and laws. Thus, by reading and interpreting these transindividual inscriptions, an individual is involved in a transindividual individuation and becomes a citizen. However, this exteriorization doesn't necessarily lead to the creation of a citizen figure; it could also lead to disindividuation, which creates the figure of the proletariat. As Read points out, "Stiegler's 'proletariat' [...] is not a class with nothing to lose but its chains, rather it is a class that has always already lost its fundamental knowledge, activity and individuation" (Read 2016: 187–88). Proletarianization means that the work is done mechanically, and the skills and knowledge are externalised into the machine. The loss of knowledge is the loss of individuation because the externalised knowledge cannot be internalised and thus cannot become the basis for new individuations.

And yet, Stiegler's interpretation of the transindividual raises some methodological questions. First, Stiegler's interpretation of the transindividual is related only to cultural human-created artefacts and thus ignores the creativity of natural objects and nature. Stiegler does not take into account the creativity of natural objects as Simondon does: as mentioned earlier, for Simondon, the transindividual means a relationship with pre-individual potential, which generally designates nature. Here, we can recall the role of the river in the functioning of the Guimbal turbine: the river as a natural force is a necessary component of technical invention. The Guimbal turbine functions only through collaboration with the river, which has the potential to produce energy and heat and also has the potential to cool it down. In this case, we have a natural object (a river), a technical object (a turbine), and a human inventor who, through her invention, is related to all other individuals (the collective). This means that not every technical object can create a transindividual relationship; it is transindividual only in the sense that it contains some tension or metastability, which is resolved by introducing a human invention. For Stiegler, this metastable pre-individual condition is lost, and the initiative is given to the human consumer: the citizen is the knowledgeable consumer who is engaged in a dialogue with memory and history, whereas the proletariat lacks both knowledge and skills and is unable to interact with technical and cultural objects.

Second, Stiegler's notion of the transindividual is so closely attached to the intergenerational past (technological memory as tertiary retention) that it risks becoming a museum of everything. The problem here is how to avoid the museumification of the past and its normative and prescriptive imperative. As Yuk Hui points out, what is missing in Stiegler's scheme is the concept of "tertiary protention," which would allow us to anticipate and imagine the most probable future. Tertiary retention means memories that are stored in technological prostheses, whereas tertiary protention means the prediction of the future that is delegated to algorithmic calculations. Tertiary protention is posthuman in the sense that it refers to the future, which wouldn't be just our future but could be the future of other generations or even other species. Stiegler does not take into account this futuristic dimension of transindividuality; however, he admits that there is a recursive causality between tertiary retentions – historical technologies and artefacts – and the capacity to imagine or predict future developments.

4 The Transindividual as a New Mode of Community?

Now, having these different interpretations of the transindividual in mind, we can ask what it means for a community and how it deals with power relationships. Can we imagine a transindividual community that is in contact with some pre-individual potential and, at the same time, can share this pre-individual potential with other members of the community by inventing new lines of individuation? Can we think about new forms of biopolitics that would relate not only to human individuals but also would connect human individuals and nonhuman entities? In other words, can we extend biopolitics into cosmopolitics?

To investigate this new area of thinking, I want to make several suggestions. What specific examples could reveal the relationships between the pre-individual (natural) potential and human individuals who could create collective individuations in one way or another? The first example I would like to consider is nuclear waste. Radioactivity is a natural element that can be potentially useful or harmful depending on human manipulation. It can create large amounts of (relatively clean) energy, and it also can be lethal when transformed into a nuclear weapon or if the nuclear power plant is damaged by natural or human causes. In the case of nuclear disasters, radioactivity penetrates not only the bodies of contemporaries but also leaves its traces for many generations to come. Knowing that nuclear waste will be radioactive for 100,000 years after its deactivation, we can ask what kind of transindividual collective it creates for the future. The radioactive waste left by such disasters as Chernobyl connects communities of those who have died and those who survived, and it also creates – in a preemptive way – future collectives of those who will have to deal with the material consequences of this event. Together with Slavoj Žižek, who argued that the Chernobyl catastrophe was the event that triggered the end of Soviet Communism (Žižek 2020: 39), we can speculate what kind of transindividual collective it might create in the future.

Another example is the recent COVID-19 pandemic, which makes us think about the role of viruses as a certain pre-individual potential. Viruses are potential in the sense that they can have different effects: they can be dangerous and lethal, but, on the other hand, there is some evidence that viruses have actively participated in the evolution of life forms. As Katherine Hayles points out, "Recent research is accumulating evidence that virus-like elements may have catalyzed some of life's critical stages, including the evolution of DNA, the formation of the first cells, and the evolutionary split into the three domains of Archaea, bacteria, and eukaryotes" (Hayles 2021: S71). Viruses are participating not only in the evolution of life forms but also are active in human embryonic stem cells. "Stem cells are crucial to human reproduction because they are pluripotent, having the ability to transform into all the different kinds of cells in the body as the fetus grows. Recent studies have found that one class of endogenous retroviruses, known as H. HERV-H, has DNA that is active in human embryonic stem cells but not in other types of human cells. (...) Without the pluripotency provided by stem cells, human reproduction could not work. Ironically then, the viral contamination that is posing a deadly threat to contemporary humans is also, in another guise, critical for human reproduction" (Hayles 2021: S71). As Hayles explains, viruses are actively participating in human reproduction; thus, there is no strict opposition between humans and viruses. We have to rethink in what ways we are interconnected with other life forms and what consequences this awareness has for us, humans.

In his recent article, Balibar is reflecting on the COVID-19 pandemic as a biopolitical condition, which reveals something new in the ontological status of the human species. A virus that is a limit-case in the classification of the living not only circulates between human individuals but also crosses the species barrier between humans and nonhumans. In this respect, humans and viruses are unified in a "passive synthesis" and create a transindividual condition. As Balibar points out, "This is a phenomenon of *trans-individuation* of the human, whose specific conditions lie both at the *pre-individual* level of the pathogenic circulation of viruses, which connect bodies and cross every frontier despite the prophylactic obstacles, and at the *supra-individual* level, formed by the 'global' system of production and communications, the *institutional* circulation of persons and things" (Balibar 2021a: 3). Balibar here directly refers to Simondon's notion of the transindividual and argues that the pandemic condition creates new forms of transindividuality where human individuals are united and unified (although negatively, through illness and death) and, at the same time, are differentiated. These are "anthropological differences" of race, gender, age, pre-existing pathologies, and "class differences," referring to jobs, revenues, precariousness, housing, access to medical services, etc., and also global geographic inequalities related to the history of colonization (Balibar 2021a: 4). All kinds of differences work to create biopolitical divisions or sub-species within the human species; however, even if these biopolitical measures are still in power, we can see the emergence of transindividual biopolitics which unifies everyone as a specimen of the human species. This transformation of humanity into the human species is a specific condition where "the human species has practically 'crossed' every species barrier technically or biologically, but, in 'doing' this (…) it has created the conditions for its *own 'barrier' as a species* to be crossed by certain organisms or quasi-organisms (such as viruses)" (Balibar 2021a: 9). This means that besides "conventional biopolitics" which is still in power and which discriminates between different sub-species, we can discern a transindividual biopolitics whose field of operation is not an individual, or a group, but the human species as such formed from human alliances with nonhuman viruses.

If viruses (with their capacity to augment and diminish life) represent the pre-individual potential, vaccination represents the technological part of this transindividual condition. In times of pandemic, individual immunity cannot be achieved without this transindividual condition, where every vaccinated individual is protecting not only their own life but also the lives of other individuals. The attempt to create a collective immunity (or so-called "herd immunity") can be seen as a new transindividual condition, where every individual is confronted with the pre-individual (namely, a virus) and, at the same time, with other individuals with whom it shares its collective immunity. A phenomenon of "common immunity" is a good example of transindividuality where a human-invented technology (a mRNA vaccine) intervenes in every individual to make collective existence possible. The transindividual here means the exteriorization of an individual, their folding out, and, at the same time, their commonality with other individuals created through technical inventiveness. Vaccination is also preemptive in the sense that it creates the conditions for future immunity. Using Stiegler's terminology, we can say that vaccination is a technology that functions in a mode of tertiary protention: it is capable not only of evaluating present health conditions but also of anticipating and predicting immunity in the future. As Yuk Hui points out, the pre-emption of the tertiary protention is possible only because of technological recursivity: "It constantly evaluates the past in order to anticipate the future, which in turn determines the present. Human beings are reintegrated into the temporality of machines, not only as individuals but also as collectives and communities" (Hui 2019: 243). On the one hand, this can be interpreted as technological or algorithmic governance, usually seen as a threat to human freedom; on the other hand, it can be seen as a life-saving condition not only to individuals but also to the entire human species.

These examples of transindividual conditions, one related to nuclear waste and another to the pandemic (and this list could be extended by including other substances, for example, plastic waste, sugar, or carbon dioxide), make us qualify the transindividual as an important biopolitical category. Taking into account the transindividual condition, Balibar (2021b) argues that although the notion of biopolitics is still relevant (to the extent that differentiation of individuals never disappears), it has to be supplemented with the notion of cosmopolitics: cosmopolitics here refers not to someone free from national prejudices but someone entangled with pre-individual potential and supra-individual technologies. Inspired by Dipesh Chakrabarty's (2009; 2021) ideas that human history cannot be examined separately from geological history and the history of industrialization, Balibar argues that recent challenges, such as the pandemic or climate change, force us to take into account the larger picture and reconsider the cosmopolitical dimension. As Chakrabarty points out, the human figure has doubled: "There was (and still is) the human of humanist histories – the human capable of struggling for equality and fairness among other humans while caring for the environment and certain forms of nonhuman life. And then there was this other human, the human as a geological agent, whose history could not be recounted from within purely humanocentric views" (Chakrabarty 2021: 3). This means that it is not enough to examine human history; another dimension has to be added – that of geological timescales. Human beings are manipulating the environment to such an extent that humanity becomes a planetary geological agent. Thus, human politics has to be complemented by planetary biopolitics that would include the geological timescale of deep history.

This geological dimension leads us to the question of the Anthropocene and makes us wonder to what extent climate change is a transindividual condition. As Chakrabarty points out, the geological time scale gives us a glimpse into the conjoined histories: the history of the planet (which is the object of Earth System Science), the history of biological life, including human life, and the history of technological development (Chakrabarty 2021: 49). The entanglements between these histories produce a new transindividual condition – that of the Anthropocene. The Anthropocene introduces humans to a geological timescale which is beyond human comprehension and reach. This geological timescale raises the question of habitability, which references not only humans but life in general and makes us rethink the question of biopolitics. "The problem of habitability therefore should be distinguished from the discussion on life that has gone on in the humanities under the rubric of biopolitics. The idea of biopolitics that connects life to questions of disciplinary power, state, capitalism, and so on and rejects 'a biological or metaphysical thematization of life' would squarely be a part of what I have characterized here as global thought" (Chakrabarty 2021: 83). If the planet is to become not habitable, we would have a world without humans and complex life, and, therefore, without biopolitics. So, if we take into account this planetary (Chakrabarty) or cosmopolitical (Balibar) dimension, we realize that human life takes only a short period between tertiary retentions (memories retained in the machines) and tertiary protentions (predictions generated by machines). This is our new transindividual or cosmopolitical condition.

On the one hand, there is some danger that this technological alienation might create an effect of anaesthetization and somehow put aside the question of responsibility. On the other hand, human responsibility does not disappear; therefore, it is important to maintain a biopolitical dimension. As Chakrabarty points out, "Humans cannot afford to give up on the political [...], but we need to resituate it within the awareness of a predicament that now marks the human condition. Political thought has so far been humanocentric, holding constant the 'world' outside of human concerns or treating its eruptions into the time of human history as intrusions from the 'outside.' This 'outside' no longer exists" (Chakrabarty 2021: 178). From now on, politics should take into consideration biopolitical differences and also reflect the cosmopolitical entanglements of human life with geo-biochemical processes of the planet.

5 Conclusion

Thus, Simondon proposes a new approach to collective existence, which includes some pre-individual potential, human individual, and human-invented technology. What interests us is the transindividual condition, and the COVID-19 pandemic is seen as one of many possible examples of such a collective mode of existence. The attempt to create a collective immunity (or "herd immunity") can be seen as a transindividual condition, where every individual is confronted with something pre-individual (namely, a virus) and, at the same time, with other individuals with whom it shares its immunity, thus creating a relationship of responsibility and solidarity. This example of transindividuality can be reconsidered as a new mode of biopolitics, conceptualized not as a negative force but as an affirmative transindividual interaction between human and nonhuman forces. Such reconceptualization of biopolitics would change the focus from the opposition between a malicious sovereign and subjugated individuals to the affirmative model of transindividual communities. To summarize, I would argue that (1) biopolitics should focus not on the deeds of some malicious sovereign power manipulating everything around it but on the formation of transindividual collectives; (2) biopolitics should detach itself from the anthropocentric model and embrace biological and geo-biochemical conditions of the planet and the geological timescale of deep time; in other words, biopolitics should be coupled with cosmopolitics; (3) biopolitics should be enlarged in such a way as to include both technical objects and technological environments; it should open itself to transindividual forms of temporality, including both tertiary retentions of past generations, and the preemptive forms of tertiary protentions, such as anticipation, invention, and imagination.

References

Agamben, G. 2021. *Where Are We Now? The Epidemic as Politics*, translated by Valeria Dani. London: Eris.

Balibar, E. 2020. *Spinoza, the Transindividual*, translated by Mark G. E. Kelly. Edinburgh: Edinburgh University Press.

Balibar, E. 2021a. "Human Species as Biopolitical Concept", *Radical Philosophy* 211, Winter, pp. 3–12.

Balibar, E. 2021b. "One World, One Health, One Species? Cosmopolitics in the Pandemic." Recording from 30th June 2021, the Birkbeck Institute for the Humanities, https://www.youtube.com/watch?v=tLzCYo6QhhA. Accessed 5 February 2024.

Braidotti, R. 2020. "We" Are In *This* Together, But We Are Not One and the Same", *Bioethical Inquiry*, https://doi.org/10.1007/s11673-020-10017-8. Accessed 5 February 2024.

Chakrabarty, D. 2009. "The Climate of History: Four Theses", *Critical Inquiry*, 35(2): pp. 197–222.

Chakrabarty, D. 2021. *The Climate of History in a Planetary Age*. Chicago and London: The University of Chicago Press.

Combes, M. 2013. *Gilbert Simondon and the Philosophy of the Transindividual*, translated by Thomas LaMarre. Cambridge, Mass: The MIT Press.

Hayles, N. K. 2021. "Novel Corona: Posthuman Virus", *Critical Inquiry*, Vol. 47 (Winter 2021), p. S68–S72, https://www.journals.uchicago.edu/doi/10.1086/711439. Accessed 5 February 2024.

Hui, Y. 2019. *Recursivity and Contingency*, London and New York: Rowman and Littlefield.

Read, J. 2016. *The Politics of Transindividuality*. Chicago: Haymarket Books.

Simondon, G. 2017. *On the Mode of Existence of Technical Objects*, translated by Cécile Malaspina and John Rogove, Minneapolis: Univocal Publishing.

Simondon, G. 2020. *Individuation in Light of Notions of Form and Information*, translated by Taylor Adkins. Minneapolis: University of Minnesota Press.

Stiegler, B. 1998. *Technics and Time, 1: The Fault of Epimetheus*, translated by Richard Beardsworth and George Collins, Stanford: Stanford University Press.

Žižek, S. 2020. *PANDEMIC! COVID-19 Shakes the World*. New York, London: OR Books.

CHAPTER 7

Post-pandemic Biopolitics: Reconciling the Geological, the Global, and the Planetary

Aistis Žekevičius

Abstract

This chapter questions the viability of biopolitics in post-pandemic times, underscoring the urgency of adopting a new biopolitical paradigm that transcends anthropocentrism and acknowledges the interconnectedness of both human and non-human life. First, it delves into a complex interplay between the grammar of geology and biopolitics within the context of the Anthropocene to establish a broader understanding of race as extending beyond biological distinctions to encompass culturally determined differences, influencing socio-cultural dynamics. Second, the chapter calls for a reevaluation of political institutions and governance structures in the face of planetary crises, urging humanity to move beyond the legacies of modernity and embrace a more holistic approach to sustainability, encompassing care for the biosphere. Last but not least, it acknowledges the urgency of extending the right to live beyond human beings and changing relationships with the environment while at the same time highlighting the uncertainties and complexities involved in establishing equitable and realistic planetary biopolitics.

Keywords

biopolitics – geology – pandemic – the global – the planetary

1 Introduction

In March 2020, as countries around the world began closing their borders and planes started abandoning the airspace due to the lockdown imposed in the hope of curbing the spread of the pandemic, it already seemed questionable that even the strictest measures to prevent the dissemination of the deadly virus, such as temporary isolation of entire countries and a (nearly) global quarantine, would suffice to ensure the liveability of planetary multitudes.

 | DOI:10.1163/9789004748187_009

After the pandemic, however, it is clear that the "think globally, act locally" paradigm turned out to be largely ineffective in the fight against COVID-19, as the inseparability of the latent logic of race and biopolitics, distinguished by the prevalence of differential vulnerability, has exposed the intensification of racial inequalities and the ensuing dissipation of entire populations, caused mainly by various complications of the virus. Indeed, the perception of the centrality of the human species in the evolution of Earth has been with us for more than three decades now (Woodhouse 1988), and the notion of planetary health, while still deeply rooted in anthropocentric thinking,[1] has preceded the COVID-19 pandemic.

One could expect that the status quo has notably shifted since the emergence of the planetary turn paradigm, which originated as an attempt to move away from the totalizing nature of globalization and signified the rise of the critical-theoretical model of planetarity[2] (Elias and Moraru 2015). Unfortunately, a lack of genuine planetary thinking, "one that takes the planetary as its own condition and exposes its limits" (Hui 2020: 868), considers not only the world's populations but also entire ecosystems consisting of hundreds of species, persists not only in the practical realm of everyday politics but also in the dominant discourse of biopolitical theory. One of the few notable exceptions, though, has been Miguel Vatter, who has recently argued for the centrality of the notion of habitability in planetary governmentality (Vatter 2022). However, most researchers still treat biopolitical interactions as part and parcel of the global and not the planetary framework. These factors allow one to raise a series of questions regarding the post-pandemic condition in terms of the viability of biopolitics in post-pandemic times. Can one honestly speak of the universality of liveability today? If so, what kind of mechanisms ensure that the shares of liveability are equally distributed on the planetary level? Is the idea of planetary biopolitics, based on thinking in non-human scales, applicable at all in terms of theory and practice of the post-pandemic condition?

1 Walton defines planetary health as "the health of human civilisation and the state of the natural system on which it depends," thereby following the long-standing tradition of placing culture above nature in the implicit yet obvious hierarchy (Walton 2019: 14).

2 It is important to note that the discourse of planetarity itself is largely of phenomenological nature, as it presents itself first and foremost "as a new *structure of awareness*, as a methodical receptivity to the *geothematics of planetariness* characteristic of a fast-expanding series of cultural formations" (emphasis by authors) (Elias and Moraru 2015: xi-xii). Oddly enough, Chakrabarty makes no mention of Elias and Moraru in none of his later works on the interplay between the global and the planetary, even though they were the first to juxtapose the two.

To address these troubling yet timely questions, I am revisiting a number of contemporary postcolonial and biopolitical theories, presenting their critical analysis, and applying a few modifications to them to suggest that an effective analysis of post-pandemic biopolitics should by no means stick to one of the paradigms that are discussed in the chapter – the geological, the global, or the planetary – but rather integrate certain aspects from each of them. In order to do so, I start with the analysis of Kathryn Yusoff's geological critique of Anthropocene and Dipesh Chakrabarty's revision of Anthropocene, with the former highlighting the material and colonial nature of Anthropocene and the latter drawing upon the distinction between the human and the natural to juxtapose the global and the planetary epistemes. Later, I turn to Achille Mbembe's negative planetary biopolitics, based on the critique of structural-inequality-laden planetary mega processes, and end by focusing on Benjamin H. Bratton's theory of positive planetary biopolitics, all the while questioning its future viability. Finally, I propose a brief outline of the notion of geoplanetary biopolitics to address the insufficiencies in adequately assessing the role of race and racialization in biopolitics.

2 Bridging the Spatial and the Temporal: Applying the Grammar of Geology to Form New Philosophical Anthropologies

The idea that the logic of race is by no means limited within the confines of local manifestations of racism and is operating not only in the area of biological distinctions but also in the sphere of culturally determined differences has already been proposed by a number of researchers who have largely focused on racialization and its socio-cultural consequences (Anthias, Yuval-Davis 1993; Fields, Fields 2012; Malik 1996; Miles 2000; Miles et Brown 2003; Murji, Solomos 2005; Weinbaum 2019). However, if we agree that the logic of race unfolds not only on the biological but also on the cultural level, one suspects that the processual understanding of race is by no means limited to the diachronic dimension but also covers both spatiality and temporality of biopolitics. This becomes especially relevant when employing planetary thinking, imbued with awareness that geography overlaps with geology, as one careless flap of butterfly wings in a Brazilian rainforest can send ripples throughout the entire Northern Hemisphere.

These suspicions are somewhat confirmed by Kathryn Yusoff, a British expert on inhuman geography. In her most renowned book, *A Billion Black Anthropocenes, or None*, Yusoff offers an exercise in "geological recasting of historical time" (Mbembe 2021b: 222) and examines the racial prehistory of the Anthropocene by emphasizing the role of geology in the continuum of liberal subjectivity and the inevitable historicity of the latter while criticizing the abandonment (or at least avoidance) of the category of race as seen in the works of most of the thinkers of Anthropocene. Referring to the historical connections between the emergence of modern liberalism and colonial coercion, on the one hand, and the ideas of freedom and the apparatus of slavery, on the other, Yusoff criticizes the dominant discourse of the Anthropocene based on "a geophysics of anti-Blackness," guided by a universalist conception of geology, cloaked in specific markers of geological time (such as the Industrial Revolution or the Great Acceleration), and yet unable (and/or unwilling) to recognize its implications for shaping the present and the future (Yusoff 2018: 110). Such discourse not only ignores but even covers up histories of racism based on oppression, coercion, and the expropriation of property rights that flourished in the regulatory structure of geological relations, while at the same time consolidating its power through the naturalization and neutralization of these histories, geological infrastructure (material political economy, including mines, pipelines, rights to water, etc.), and the imposition of a racialized view (Yusoff 2018: 22–23, 33–34). Yet what is perhaps the most innovative in Yusoff's philosophy is the attempt to organically combine the material and discursive planes while rethinking the axis of power and exploitation, which overlaps geological features and the narratives on human history provided by them.

While criticizing the tendency to overcome the colonial legacy without rejecting its symbolic discursive power, Yusoff links the birth of the racial categorization of blackness to the origins of the New World resource mining, thereby highlighting the historical connections of the categories of the human and the inhuman to the settler-colonialist rights discourse and material extraction practices, referred to as the categorization of matter. What lies beneath this umbrella category? Yusoff provides a processual definition of the categorization of matter: it is the spatial destruction of active and inert, activated and passive, corporeal and mineralogical matter – individuals and natural resources – by detaching this matter from geography and relocating it through indentured servitude and transatlantic slavery, thereby destroying the fabric that binds this matter – the relational network. To identify such matter, a certain epistemic act is necessary, during which the inhumanity of the exploitation of this matter is recognized and acknowledged (Yusoff 2018: 14). Furthermore, Yusoff notes that the reterritorialization of the inhumane, conceived of as a geopoetic resource, allows for a better understanding of the functioning of material divisions since it is precisely the distinction between the "dead matter" and the privileged "live subject," between those who can become subjects and those who cannot, which establishes an active politics of recognition in the late liberalism (Yusoff 2018: 62–63, 65). At first glance, it may seem unclear how Yusoff's reformulation of the concept of matter contributes to the discussion of planetary biopolitics. However, it soon becomes clear that the author does not see the possibility of agreeing on a new planetary language guided by biopolitical regimes of inclusion due to the hierarchical differences that distinguish the biocentric subject, located at the very core of these regimes, and associates the birth of the racial subject with colonialism, the conquest of space, and the codification of geology as both property and properties.

In her most recent monograph, *Geologic Life: Inhuman Intimacies and the Geophysics of Race*, Yusoff overtly claims that race, rather than being a biocentric or biopolitical concept, is first and foremost a geologic and geopolitical formation (Yusoff 2024: 4, 10). Therefore, race should be considered primarily as a geophysical operation and not as a core element of biopolitics; for Yusoff, it would be "a mistake to understand race as a biopolitical concept when it is materially and conceptually grounded in the earth in advance, and the focus on *bios* covers over the racial deficit of the spatial extractions underway" (Yusoff 2024: 12–13). Such a theoretical perspective, based on a clear preference for material rather than relational aspects of racialization, allows her to formulate a materialist version of bio-, or rather, geo-politics of race where race is no less a geological than a biological factor. Refusing to accept the division between *geos* and *bios* she sees as false and inhuman, Yusoff highlights the modulating and mediating role of race in maintaining this division, on the one hand, and the production of racialized life and reproduction of "the geo-logic of extraction" as effects of that division, which functions as a standalone instrument of (geo)power, on the other.

Although the inclusion of such *geologic grammars* in the analysis of the interplay between biopolitics and race may appear questionable at first, Yusoff sees geology as nothing less than "a mechanism of power and statecraft that has a lower resolution or a more subterranean subjective operation than the more performative biopolitics" in terms of extractive properties and leaving sediments in colonial states, which "nonetheless continues to be repressive in its extraction qualities and sediments the settler-colonial state" and argues for establishing a biopolitical difference between descriptions of geology and its corporeal affects, which produce a "monstrous impolitic materiality," whose one of the most detrimental effects is the inception of an instrumental relationship with the land, ecology, and people (Yusoff 2018: 86–87). By emphasizing the colonial origins of geology and treating it as a classificatory regime that contextualizes the emergence of the privileged biocentric subject, Yusoff brings attention to the historical links between geology and racialization processes via the discourse of speciesism and progress. Finally, Yusoff observes that the discipline of geology has long functioned as a practice that inscribes the logic of race into the material politics of extraction and establishes living forms of racism, ranging from eugenics to environmental racism, and that the science of geology, concerned with the organization and categorization of matter, institutes not only colonial practices but also a certain taxonomy of race, which generates a logic of race extending far beyond mineralogy, linking geological formations and perceptions of social structures (Yusoff 2018: 86). And while geology itself does not produce or reproduce race as such, geological claims are inseparable from claims of racial identity, as both participate in empirical processes equating nonhuman property with racial codification. Furthermore, in assuming what is worth explaining about slavery and what is not, a geohistorical horizon is being drawn, in which issues of race and opportunity are taken as differentiated in time, thereby justifying slavery and the material expropriation of property (Yusoff 2018: 79, 83). Yusoff emphasizes the role of race in defining the inhuman, especially the transition from inhuman matter to inhuman race, examining the inhuman as the link between the paradoxically related discourses of geology and humanism and establishing an axis based on unrestrained extraction of both the subject and the geological sphere. This becomes particularly evident when one turns to the category of corporeality, equated with territoriality expressed in relation to black subjects, starting from plantation slavery and ending with the contemporary environmental racism, in which blackness becomes what Yusoff calls "an ontology without territory" – a will-less, deterritorialized, and racialized matter, distinguished by the prevalence of grammars of extraction (Yusoff 2018: 87–90). Finally, Yusoff associates the logic of race with fossil narratives, racialized extraction processes, and modes of racial discourse that are inseparable from the ideas of wealth, property, and land use. In categorizing matter into property and properties via the spatial dispossession of land for extractive purposes and the slavish dispossession of personal rights, the slave is reformulated as matter and recognized through inhuman property relations "as a commodity with properties, but without subjective will or agency" (Yusoff 2018: 16–17). Yet ultimately, it is the conception of the subject as inhuman matter that incorporates the historical fact of the extraction of individual rights into the concept of geology.

What solutions, if any, are offered by Yusoff as a counterpoint to the conception of the subject as inhuman matter? She proposes a project called *a billion black Anthropocenes* that is based on the reconfiguration of the subject by writing colonial history into the Anthropocene and recognizing the role of race in producing humanity, which brings to the surface the violent shadow of geology, considered by Yusoff as a formation that consists not only of materiality but also of time. The aim of Yusoff's project is simple – to dissolve any illusions about the neutrality of the Anthropocene and the role of race in its formation by reconsidering the territorial implications of geological forces and their subjective regimes, on the one hand, and inscribing in the geological event the appropriate symbolic connection with the translation of matter and specific spatial practices based on the logic of race, on the other (Yusoff 2018: 67–68). Furthermore, Yusoff's subject is nothing more than an inhuman (or rather a dehumanized) object, localized beyond human experience and thus placed beyond the category of human (Yusoff 2018: 64). Yet what lies at the very heart of her project is the desire to deny the newness of the Anthropocene, as the researcher traces the historical continuity of its processes, starting with the first slaves brought from Africa to the Americas at the end of the fifteenth century, and ending with contemporary subjects trapped in a landscape of tightening geopolitical boundaries and material destratification, thereby refusing to focus solely on planetary-scale modernity or human failures while the colonial nature of the Anthropocene remains on the sidelines (Yusoff 2018: 67–69). Ultimately, the idea of a billion black Anthropocenes, proposed by Yusoff, rejects the structural whiteness of the Anthropocene that is grounded in unequal power relations, and acts as a necessary condition for rewriting the origin story of the Anthropocene, thereby replacing it with a new geology centred on racialized assemblages and responsible for creating more accountable, decolonized, and geosocial – and, one may add, geo-solidary – futures.

While Yusoff, as already noted, is not particularly concerned about the possible impact of her grammar of geology on the dominant formulations of biopolitics, some of the work regarding geological structures of the planet and reformulating biopolitics has already been done by American anthropologist Elizabeth A. Povinelli. In one of her more recent works, *Geontologies: A Requiem to Late Liberalism*, Povinelli coins the term geontological power, or *geontopower*, challenging the classical biopolitical distinction between life and nonlife, supported by proponents of biopower, which she defies as "the governance of life and the tactics of death," and thereby intensifying the paradox that sees nonlife (*geos*) and being (ontology) working in unison (Povinelli 2016: 4–5; emphasis by author). For Povinelli, geontopower functions primarily as a deconstructive force whose main purpose is shining light on the figural tactics of late liberalism as a long-standing biontological orientation and distribution of power. She criticizes the continuous use of the language of sovereignty, disciplinary power, and biopolitics as if these formations were independent of each other and of history. And while each of these power formations has its own expression and tactics, one cannot shake off an impression that there is a certain unnamed common conceptual matrix that binds them all together. Povinelli, then, connects this conceptual matrix with an ontological claim that there is a distinction between Life and Nonlife, which becomes questionable in the context of posthumanism and Anthropocene theories, since *anthropos* becomes only one of many elements in the realm of vitalistic Life, conceived of as opposed to the inert state of Nonlife. In turn, this also determines a certain ontological fragility of *anthropos*, since it remains in the matrix of Life only as long as Life is able to maintain the distinction from Death/Extinction and Nonlife. Therefore, the strategies of late liberalism, structuring the management not only of markets but also of any differences, can only work if this fundamental distinction is maintained (Povinelli 2016: 7–9). In other words, Povinelli no longer sees any point in adhering to the traditional anthropocentric model of biopolitics, which was promoted by the authors of conventional biopolitical theories, not only because of a certain indifference of this paradigm to the plane of material history but also due to the latter's inability to respond to changes of planetary scale, which necessitate a rethinking of the boundaries of ontology itself. Following Povinelli, it can be argued that in the context of racial categorization, in which established populations constantly balance on the edge of Death or Extinction due to their differentiated vulnerability, the boundary that separates Life and Nonlife is much more fluid than it is accustomed to think, if not questionable altogether.

The works of Dipesh Chakrabarty, an Indian post-colonial theorist, are no less significant in considering the possible ways of reimagining the Anthropocene (and no less critical regarding it). While Chakrabarty acknowledges the relative importance and effectiveness of the Anthropocene theory, he criticizes the Anthropocene's refusal to differentiate humanity (*anthropos*), even though the rich and well-to-do beneficiaries of capitalism bear far greater historical responsibility for the destruction of the planetary life support system than impoverished populations, situated on the margins of the global economy (Chakrabarty 2023a: xv). In the book *The Crises of Civilization: Exploring Global and Planetary Histories*, Chakrabarty formulates four theses about the climate of history, which allow us not only to unpack Chakrabarty's distinctive concept of the Anthropocene but also realize the connections and differences between the histories of capital and species. In short, these four theses are as follows: first, anthropogenic interpretations of climate change suggest the disappearance of the humanist distinction between natural history and human history; second, the idea of the Anthropocene as a new geological epoch in which man becomes a geological power significantly modifies humanistic narratives of modernity and globalization; third, the geological hypothesis of the Anthropocene requires the inclusion of the history of humanity as a species in dialogue with the global histories of capital; and fourth, the interweaving of the histories of species and capital allows us to expand the limits of history and its understanding (Chakrabarty 2018: 194–214). For Chakrabarty, such a conception of the climate of history allows for distinguishing between three separate histories that develop at such divergent rates that they can be considered separate processes that are taking place on different time scales: the history of the Earth system, the history of life (which also encompasses human evolution), and the history of industrial civilization.

It is here that Chakrabarty identifies one of the greatest pitfalls associated with anthropogenic climate change – to understand its scale and the duration of its consequences, one must think on both gigantic and miniature scales simultaneously (Chakrabarty 2021: 49–51). Borrowing the notion of technosphere,[3] coined by the eminent geologist Peter Haff and used to describe the global system of human technology, Chakrabarty admits that in a world where human impact on the planet's geology has surpassed other global factors in intensity, the Earth's ability to support the life of a multi-billion human population primarily depends on ensuring the smooth functioning of the technosphere on a daily basis (Chakrabarty 2021: 6). As humanity's capabilities of disrupting the natural environment have intensified, Chakrabarty sees a certain "dualization" of the human figure, brought about by the juxtaposition of modern man and geophysical power, allowing the former to be seen as both human and inhuman, an autonomous conscious actor in humanist stories and, at the same time, a depersonalized unconscious geological agent which lives in two temporal regimes, consisting of the present of human history and the present of long geological and biological durations – all notwithstanding the fact that man cannot experience and reflect himself as a geophysical power at the phenomenological level (Chakrabarty 2018: 262–263; Chakrabarty 2021: 3–7). However, despite all efforts, as anthropocentrism retains its epistemic dominance, thinking in non-human durations remains a very strenuous exercise in today's world.

3 Haff's definition of the technosphere is as follows: "the set of large-scale networked technologies that underlie and make possible rapid extraction from the Earth of large quantities of free energy and subsequent power generation, long-distance, nearly instantaneous communication, rapid long-distance energy and mass transport, the existence of modern governmental and other bureaucracies, high-intensity industrial and manufacturing operations including regional, continental and global distribution of food and other goods, and myriad additional "artificial" or "non-natural" processes without which modern civilization and its present 7 × 10 human constituents could not exist" (Haff 2014: 301–302).

Thinking of possible alternatives to anthropocentric Anthropocene, Chakrabarty offers a paradigm of enlightened anthropocentrism based on a diverse and contradictory conception of man[4] and the idea that while both the role of humanity and the scale of exploitation of nature have increased several times over the past few centuries, the health of the planet is more important than the desire to raise the well-being of humanity at all costs (Chakrabarty 2018: 241). That said, Chakrabarty is by no means the first to criticize the excessive attention to the anthropocentric approach, associated with the critique of globalization. Following the ideas of W. E. B. Du Bois, Spivak has claimed that today, we must fundamentally rethink globalization and replace it with planetarity, a concept relying not so much on *istoria* as on *teleopoiesis*.[5] While Spivak admits that thinking along planetary lines is by no means an easy task, she claims that it is easiest to do so by imagining the pre-capitalist cultures of the planet and uses the catachresis "planet" to refer to a collective commitment to developing a certain form of law based on the principle of otherness, while simultaneously taking into account other forms of life as well (Spivak 2003: 97–102). However, Chakrabarty remains sceptical of the capabilities of scientific knowledge and climate change analysis in ensuring that actual actions will be taken for the planetary good. For this reason, Chakrabarty urges us to ponder not only on globality – an anthropocentric construct based on the principles of sustainability, inseparable from the most recent history of mankind, the accompanying intensification of capitalist globalization, and the global warming crisis caused by the latter – but also on planetarity, a concept that decentralizes the human figure and is based on the concept of a dual subject and the interaction of different life forms, allowing us to recognize the human ability to intervene in planetary-scale processes, which does not necessarily coincide with the ability

4 In Chakrabarty's conception of man, man is seen "as a geophysical power and as a political agent, as a bearer of rights and as author of actions; subject to both the stochastic forces of nature (being itself one such force collectively) and open to the contingency of individual human experience; belonging at once to differently scaled histories of the planet, of life and species, and of human societies" (Chakrabarty 2018: 268).

5 A term coined by Jacques Derrida. In his philosophy, *teleiopoiós* denotes that which makes absolute, perfect, accomplished, complete, completed, that which completes. However, Scheiner notes that Spivak uses the term *teleopoiesis* in a sense that is closer to the philosophy of Gilles Deleuze, when telepoiesis is equated to copying and pasting, which should be considered production, not reproduction. This difference stems from Deleuze's distinction between repetition as simple repetition or recurrence, and repetition as addition and differentiation, during which differences are being produced, and the attention is directed towards mediation. For more information, see: Scheiner, Corinne. 2005. „Teleiopoiesis, Telepoesis, and the Practice of Comparative Literature." In: *Comparative Literature*, 57(3): 239–245.

to solve planetary-scale problems and review human history through the prism of "the inhumanly vast timescales of deep history"[6] (Chakrabarty 2021: 3–5; 81). Such amalgamation of human and non-human scales also has political implications, as any action taken to reverse climate change – starting with scientific, technological, and geoengineering experiments and ending with politics and activism of all possible ideologies – is already political, even in the absence of an all-inclusive solution because it affects the lives of many future generations (Chakrabarty 2021: 8–9). Here, it is important to realize that Chakrabarty is not suggesting to choose one of the two formats of thinking and to think only globally or only planetary; rather, he calls for an organic interrelationship between these two different mindsets, as the emergence of globality over the last seventy years, given the name of "the Great Acceleration" by an American environmental historian John McNeill, has opened up the field of planetarity to today's humanitarians and allowed planetary thinking to permeate our everyday consciousness. However, while global thinking based on ideal forms and values covers the processes that are taking place on a scale that is still perceptible to the human mind – multiple horizons of existential, intergenerational and historical time, – the planetary processes of non-human dimensions, unbound by moral imperatives, take place in completely different time intervals, some of which fit within the time limits of human experience, while the scale of others is simply unfathomable if one looks from the phenomenological standpoint (Chakrabarty 2021: 85–87). It seems that this analytical approach, based on the interaction of notions of the global and the planetary – with the planet conceived of as the Earth system, both differentiated and unitary – is most extensively discussed in the latest monograph written by Chakrabarty, *One Planet, Many Worlds: The Climate Parallax*, in which he discerns seven main differences between the globe and the planet: (1) the globe, encompassing the interaction of empires, capitalism, and technology, was created by man, conceived of as the main character in the history of the creation of the world, while the planet decentralizes man, who is deemed as having appeared too late in the geobiological history of the planet to become the main figure in the narrative; (2) the globe encompasses only the history of the recent 500 years, while the planet is based on the entire geobiological history of the planet; (3) the globe is conceived of as exclusively human and focused on human phenomenological experience, while the planet is treated as a comparative cat-

6 In the context of biopolitical research, it must be emphasized that biopolitics, known for seeing life through the lens of the disciplinary power, the state, capitalism, etc. and rejecting "a biological or metaphysical thematization of life," is unequivocally attributed to the global, and not the planetary mindset by Chakrabarty (Chakrabarty 2021: 83).

egory that presupposes interaction with other celestial bodies. However, the globe and the planet are connected by technology, which allows us to assume that we live in an age that is both global and planetary; (4) sustainability is a global and anthropocentric term, while planetarity is based on the idea of habitability; (5) global histories are written about the human-dominated order of life on this planet, while the geobiological history of the planet allows us to understand that humanity is merely a minority on a planet whose life forms are mostly microorganisms; (6) the prevailing concept of the world in modern historiography is based on the idea of the mutuality of man and his earthly environment, while the life-sustaining processes of the planet are not oriented towards man; (7) the world shaped by human institutions and technologies is susceptible to moral and political questions, and planetary-level forces are capable of reducing all political considerations to the question of survival (Chakrabarty 2023b: 4–6, 12). Finally, Chakrabarty notes that the planetary ecological crisis calls for expanding ideas of politics and justice beyond anthropocentrism to include both animate and inanimate nature and to rethink what he himself once called "political modernity," as the human condition has irreversibly changed in the Anthropocene. These days, humanity is not only a fragmented population of humans but also the driving force of a gigantic techno-socio-economic-biological complex, which also includes representatives of multiple other species. This, however, does not mean that the concepts of man as a cell of society, a representative of a species, and a geological factor can be merged into a coherent geohistory, because man cannot directly experience other modes of being, which are cognizable only at the cognitive level of abstractions (Chakrabarty 2021: 13–15). And this is precisely the reason why Chakrabarty emphasizes the importance of maintaining analytical distinctions between these interrelated categories.

What alternatives to the current political order does Chakrabarty see? Chakrabarty associates possible substitutes to the existing (bio)political order primarily with the establishment of a new philosophical paradigm. For him, any politics capable of addressing the planetary crisis that humanity is facing today must be grounded in a new philosophical anthropology based on "a new understanding of the changing place of humans in the web of life and in the connected but different histories of the globe and the planet" (Chakrabarty 2021: 91). What kind of change in mental structures or epistemic paradigms could ensure the realization of this new philosophical anthropology? In Chakrabarty's view, the first step is abandoning the attachment to classical concepts and definitions of politics, which presuppose or at least imply human domination of Earth's ecosystems, daring to think on a geobiological level, and rethinking political thought, which until now has been anthropocentric and conceived of the "world's" intrusions into human time as "external" invasions. The second, far more complex and challenging task is to learn to live simultaneously in two present times, integrating both the vast scale of geobiological time and the phenomenologically limited affective structures of human historical time and realizing that the slow climate change on the scale of planetary history is nearly instantaneous when viewed on the scale of human and world history (Chakrabarty 2021: 178–179). The third – to follow Karl Jaspers – is to adopt a certain *epochal consciousness*,[7] an ethical position that requires coming to terms, and rather stoically, with the idea that we are all living in flux, a process that fosters the understanding of a two-way relation between changes in knowledge and changes in life, in which finding technical solutions to all complex problems is not always possible (Chakrabarty 2021: 197–198). Finally, Chakrabarty formulates three ethical principles for a just and civilized future of humanity: (1) the necessity to protect the lives and prosperity of all people; (2) the need to protect biodiversity; and (3) the urge to initiate the process of man's withdrawal from the dominant position on the planet Earth (Chakrabarty 2021: 203–204). And while these slogans sound fair and rational enough, practical capabilities regarding their implementation depend first and foremost on (bio)political decision-making processes.

While Chakrabarty refrains from a direct analysis of biopolitics, one can clearly identify his implicit doubts about the prospects of biopolitical governance in the current planetary predicament. These reservations about the future of biopolitics are particularly evident in Chakrabarty's critique of those scholars who, in the face of the planet's radical otherness, turn to the human-historical present, continuing to see the planet as an exclusively human concern, while "the governance question, whether posed in terms of sustainability or habitability, is at base an existential concern that can only belong to the present" (Chakrabarty 2021: 87). At the same time, when facing planetary reality, one must admit that the communicative setup, in which people have naturally assigned themselves a place with the help of such categories as Earth, the world, and the globe, is at least partially defunct and requires new points of reference, as planetary thinking equates man with all other living beings (Chakrabarty 2021: 90). Chakrabarty also criticizes the excessive focus of political philosophy on the individual, which has indirectly led to a prevalence of an indifference to the total size of human populations, which has translated into a

7 Chakrabarty borrows the term from the German philosopher Karl Jaspers, who associates its conception with the separation of life and knowledge of life and the ensuing realization that each generation exists in "what is but a historically determined and changing situation" (Jaspers 2010: 10), solving a different set of problems concerning the situation of mankind. For more information, see: Jaspers, Karl. 2010. *Man in the Modern Age*. Oxon: Routledge.

corresponding indifference to the biosphere, thanks to which we are faced with a paradoxical situation where "the harder we "work" the earth in pursuit of the worldly flourishing of a great number of humans, the more we encounter the planet" (Chakrabarty 2021: 90–91). Thus, Chakrabarty diagnoses the weakness of political institutions and (bio)political governance in general in the face of the planetary crisis, as the political institutions, which theoretically should have ensured the liveability of humanity, have reached such a point where they themselves have begun to sabotage this aspiration, originally inseparable from their purpose. In this case, finding counterarguments to Chakrabarty is rather a daunting task, as the question of how much sense it makes to strive for sustainability in a paradigm that is based on global capitalism, when planetary-scale climatological phenomena force us to care about survival instead of raising questions of moral and political philosophy, largely remains open.

Bearing in mind that humanity has already learned to live simultaneously in two separate worlds – physical and virtual – it seems increasingly likely that living in two different time regimes will become a reality in the near future – of course, if humanity manages to learn the lessons of globalization and, if one was to paraphrase Bruno Latour, "stop being modern" – at least in the sense of thinking about the surrounding world as human-made and getting rid of the political and ideological legacies of modernity, which appear to be of no help in solving today's climatological challenges, largely caused by a reckless behaviour of our species (Latour 1993). But how long can humanity maintain the façade that the artificial distinction between culture and nature, between the human and the natural worlds, provides? With time quickly ticking away, we remain in dire need of a new biopolitical paradigm that would maintain the ethical dimension of care for human populations without excluding the rest of the biosphere.

3 Planetary Biopolitics: From a Critique of Mega Processes to a Theory of Automated Biogovernance

In the light of Yusoff's and Chakrabarty's considerations, the need for a new biopolitical paradigm emerges, one that would preserve the ethical dimension of concern for human populations, but at the same time would not distance itself from the questions regarding the Earth's biosphere and its reservoirs of life. However, before delving into the nuances of planetary biopolitics in further detail, it seems appropriate to discuss the concept of planetarity itself, even if for a moment. French philosopher Frédéric Neyrat distinguishes between two distinct dimensions of what he calls *the planetary*, consisting of *the environmental situation*, thus emphasizing the interconnectedness of each terrestrial entity and the resulting relational ontology, and *the wandering condition*, thereby highlighting the inherent separation of every terrestrial entity determined by its singularity. For Neyrat, the most challenging issue regarding the planetary is the widespread repression of our relational situation and its underlying state of wandering, which leads to the development of *planetary unconscious*, which he considers the antipode of the planetary that signifies not only a lack of planetary awareness but even a certain blindness to the planetary reality (Neyrat 2016: 40–41). Building on Neyrat's ideas, one can assume that planetary biopolitics should be characterized by a planetary awareness, based on the unconditional recognition of planetary-scale ecological challenges and the ensuing deep knowledge of planetary processes, which would allow for the prompt resolution of global problems. However, there are reasonable doubts as to whether planetary biopolitics is capable of effectively manoeuvring in the complex context of global biogovernance. Would such an approach be able to reconcile the preservation of a life-sustaining environment with economic interests? Is it truly realistic to align the theoretical principles of planetary biopolitics with the search for solutions to specific planetary-scale problems? To be better equipped to navigate these questions, I take a closer look at two versions of planetary politics, one of which is negative and the other affirmative.

The primary proponent of negative biopolitics is Achille Mbembe, who emphasizes the importance of the natural unity of humanity and the biosphere while searching for planetary solutions. In responding to the challenges of the ongoing anthropogenic climate change that equally affects both human and inhuman forms of life, Mbembe repeatedly emphasizes that to break out of the planetary impasse caused by modernity's "interminable war on life" and save the world we live in, it is crucial to realize our ecological precariousness and the vulnerability of life in order to devote ourselves to the preservation and sustenance of the reservoirs of life (Mbembe 2017: 181–182, Mbembe 2019: 176, Mbembe 2021c: S60–S62). It is by no means surprising, as Mbembe has been increasingly veering towards a theory of planetary biopolitics for a while, at least starting from the publication of his *Critique of Black Reason* in 2017. Having reframed the universal right to life as a metaphorical and literal universal right to breathe during the COVID-19 pandemic, Mbembe focuses on the threat of suffocation in the face of the planetary ecological crisis and introduces the notion of planetary combustion in his most recent texts (Mbembe 2021c, Mbembe 2024: 1–3). In his view, the main culprits of this impasse are energy-intensive resource extraction, agricultural development, predatory land acquisition, and massive deforestation. During the pandemic, we have seen videos on social media displaying people who were dealing with an actual threat of suffocation due to complications caused by the virus, ranging from shortness of breath to premature respiratory arrest (Mbembe 2021c: S60–S62). In his most recent monograph, *Brutalism*, while seemingly agreeing in principle with both Yusoff and Chakrabarty on the idea that humanity has transformed itself into a geological force, Mbembe goes as far as to announce the death of human history by arguing that "all history, including the history of power, is now, by definition, geo-history" (Mbembe 2024: xii). Such a theoretical position allows him to claim that the current era of the combustion of the world – characterized by the depletion of natural resources, toxification of food, water and air, and the inability of "the concrete time of the flesh and breath of the world" to combat the increasing intensification of time and the evacuation of duration – is nothing less than a posthistorical age, distinguished by two simultaneous processes, the becoming-artificial of humanity, and conversely, the becoming-human of objects and machines (Mbembe 2024: 1–4). And while Mbembe's claims on the posthistorical nature of today's world remain substantially contested (and he is by no means the first to declare the end of history), he validly emphasizes humanity's absolute dependence on the biosphere and the broader interconnectedness of the human and natural worlds by extending the "universal right to breathe" beyond the human realm and into nonhuman kingdoms of life, thereby bridging the biopolitical and the planetary.

Similar concerns are shared by the American poststructuralist Judith Butler, who has been criticizing the so-called *governmentality of "crisis"* and pointing out how discourses of crisis become neat tools for maintaining and "managing" bearable levels of precarity rather than functioning as solution-seeking devices long before the outbreak of the COVID-19 pandemic (Butler, Athanasiou 2013: 149–150). In her latest book, *What World Is This?* Butler recalibrates her focus on the phenomenology of the pandemic. Contemplating ecological concerns, she places the questions of the bearability of life and the liveability of the world at the centre of planetary thinking, expressing hope that revulsion and outrage caused by the racial and sexual expendability of life fulfil its revolutionary promise in the fight for the conditions for living. Borrowing the concept of the lifeworld from the Austrian-German phenomenologist Edmund Husserl, who has emphasized the importance of *Lebenswelt* to understand both our own lived experience and our impact on the surrounding world (Føllesdal 2009: 38–39), Butler emphasizes both the liveability of life and the importance of the world's habitability, two fundamental principles that shape the very core of the emerging planetary biopolitics (Butler 2022: 55). Ultimately, she claims that the category of the inhabited world is inseparable from the quality of the air we breathe and the world's favourability both for the conditions that are necessary to support life on Earth and for the preservation of the will to live, thus linking the world's habitability and the tolerability of life via an ethical prism and giving impetus to broader discussions of planetary biopolitics, and suggesting that "the lifeworlds in which we live have to be those that secure the conditions of life for all creatures whose persistence and desire to live should be equally honored" (Butler 2022: 59, 61–63). For Butler, one of the preconditions necessary to make the world life-friendly is a complete abandonment of anthropocentrism, accompanied by a conscious and tangible reduction of planetary human involvement (Butler 2022: 66). However, due to the dominance of the model of economic calculations that is based on the analysis of costs and benefits in decision-making, there are reasonable doubts regarding the factual implementation of such a policy. Butler's proposal to narrow the scope of human activity is also questionable because humanity today is intensively involved in multiple processes of the planet's biosphere and has already affected them in such a significant manner that not only the retreat itself would be complicated but also the prediction of its possible consequences would be no less unpredictable. This forces one to look for alternatives to Butler's suggestion of a return to earlier and supposedly better times, which does not appear feasible in the current post-pandemic biopolitical landscape.

What has encouraged the reconsideration of the links between biopolitics, necropolitics, and capitalism in Mbembe's most recent works? For him, some of the main culprits of the so-called planetary turn include the breakthrough in the study of the human genome, the pollution-induced imbalance of the planetary ecosystems, the inseparability of organisms and the environments in which they are living, and changes in the prevailing understanding of agency and power that allow us to attribute both agency and power to nonhuman beings, at least to some extent (Mbembe 2021a: 12–13; Mbembe 2021b: 18–19). Mbembe observes the tendency that can be characterized as movement towards a network-like entanglement of nature and society and supports his argument by identifying three main mega-processes that constitute the contemporary forms of biopower and maintain this planetary entanglement of unprecedented extent: *corporate sovereignty*, *techno-molecular colonialism*, and *the dialectics of entanglement and separation* (Mbembe 2021a: 21; Mbembe 2021b: 88). Mbembe refers to *corporate sovereignty* when taking note of the unrivalled consolidation of power and knowledge in the hands of private yet global high-tech corporations, the transformation of capitalism into a planetary financial system, and the often-underestimated social impact of financial markets. It results in the rise of their capability to monitor every single sphere of modern life, turn anything into a source of capital, reduce the Earth and all its forms of life to a financial problem, and transform life itself into a commodity and the human body into an extraction site of added value (Mbembe 2021a: 14–16, 23–24, 27–28; Mbembe 2021b: 21–23, 63). Mbembe also criticizes *techno-molecular colonialism*, or the organization of societies based on *the computational*, a *speed regime* that seeks universal algorithmization and results in the involvement of an unprecedented number of people in increasingly complex technostructures, most of which interfere with the dynamics of the Earth's system on a planetary scale (Mbembe 2021a: 16–17, 19–20, 24). It leads to two main challenges that rational thinking seems to be facing today. First, the workings of the computational reproduction of reason have obliterated its exclusivity, as reason is no longer considered the privileged domain of the human species. Second, the fusion of visual, digital, and consumer culture has transformed our relationship with reasoning and amplified calls for a rehabilitation of visceral reactions, enabling our species to prioritize affects, faith, and conviction over reason in key decision-making processes (Mbembe 2021a: 26–27; Mbembe 2021b: 23–24). Finally, Mbembe tackles *the dialectics of entanglement and separation* by taking note of a new global division into the insured and the uninsured and the ensuing redistribution of land, on the one hand, and mass migration on the other, as the symbiotic blurring of life and mobility means that being alive becomes increasingly equated with the ability to move quickly in a world where the freedom of movement is mainly reserved for privileged populations (Mbembe 2021a: 20–23; Mbembe 2021b: 31). The consequence of such a symbiotic amalgam is the creation of a segmented planet, operating at different speed regimes and based on the redistribution of life according to the criterion of the (in)surability of the body, determined by the answer to the question: can such life be insured and articulated in a concrete financial expression?

While Mbembe largely remains pessimistic about the future of humanity regarding anthropogenic climate change, he offers several recommendations that could help us save the planet. The first of these is concerned with the need to remember that the technologies of techno-molecular colonialism introduce us to only one of many possible worlds. Therefore, we can form alternative worlds by creating conditions for the appearance of new ways of seeing and computing, cultivating the alternative politics and aesthetics of being human, living on Earth, and learning to share the planet with other people and species (Mbembe 2021a: 27). The second is related to resistance to both the epistemic hegemony and the urge to reduce Earth and all life forms to a financial problem and automate society at all costs. The third solution suggests connecting the fight against racism to the ideas of human interdependence, radical sharing, and universal inclusion (Mbembe 2021a: 28; Mbembe 2021b: 20–21, 41). Finally, as an alternative to the contemporary epistemic landscape, Mbembe introduces the concept of *a planetary library*, which he sees as a relational theory of interface based on "the assumption of the inseparability of the different archives of the world" (Mbembe 2021b: 39). And yet Mbembe's approach deserves considerable criticism. His techno-pessimistic view of technological progress is not entirely groundbreaking as it builds on the ideas expressed by most theorists of automatic systems of governmentality, including Antoinette Rouvroy and Bernard Stiegler, who have extensively criticized the modelling of social reality and reorganization of psycho-power according to automatized systems (see Rouvroy, Berns, 2013; Stiegler, 2016, 2018). Also, there are substantial doubts as to whether Mbembe's highly idealistic principles are applicable to the material realm, as Mbembe offers little to nothing in terms of practical planetary-scale solutions except for the seemingly bottomless reservoirs of negativity and unwavering faith in humanistic idealism. While such a planetary approach helps to emphasize and understand the transnational aspects of biopolitics, it risks becoming too abstract, primarily because the analysis of macro-level mechanisms of biopower risks becoming overly detached from the material realities of indigenous populations, which continue to encounter biopolitics primarily at the affective level; this can also complicate the analysis of localized biopolitical practices. Finally, Mbembe's planetary biopolitics is too broad and all-encompassing. It therefore fails to take into account the interaction of global biopower structures with specific formations operating in localized contexts, which in turn limits the understanding of both the specificity of biogovernance and racialization that is inherent to it.

Another prominent representative of planetary biopolitics, Benjamin Bratton, known for putting a positive spin on it, began developing his own theory of planetary biopolitics as early as 2015 when he published *The Stack: On Software and Sovereignty*, in which he draws on political philosophy, architectural theory, and software studies to suggest that a multitude of avatars of contemporary computation form a coherent whole. Bratton sees *The Stack* as an accidental physical-informational cybernetic megastructure of planetary-scale computation, a system of systems consisting of six interconnected geologic, humanistic, and mineral layers charging feedback loops between them and distributed "under, onto, and over the surface of the globe" (Bratton 2015: 54). Later, in *The Terraforming*, Bratton develops his ideas further by identifying the main pillars of this physical-informational cybernetic megastructure: the sovereign that looks increasingly more like a technical apparatus, an artificial politics that resembles a planetary-scale geotechnology, and an artificial technology that is similar to planetary-scale geopolitics (Bratton 2019: 12). Contemplating both the current and the future ecological consequences of the Anthropocene, Bratton speaks of an urgency to reshape or *terraform* the Earth to mitigate the anthropogenic climate change and sustain life on this planet in the coming decades (Bratton 2019: 3). In his most recent work, *The Revenge of the Real: Politics for a Post-pandemic World*, Bratton rethinks biopolitics in response to three catastrophes or disasters: first, the anthropogenic climate change, second, the rapid spread of COVID-19, and third, a series of essays by Giorgio Agamben that appeared shortly after the outbreak of the pandemic.

For Bratton, the pandemic was an acute intrusion into the complex biological reality of the planet, which has revealed the anarchic nature of the current state of geopolitics, highlighting the vital need for effective planetary biopolitics, as local and international executive politics have proved to be highly anarchic and generally incapable of addressing both fundamental biopolitical problems and global challenges of governance. Calling for a new form of planetary governmentality that would encompass planetary protection, governance, and competence, Bratton advocates the implementation of new, more rational, efficient, and realistic biopolitics that would address global challenges such as climate change and pandemics through efficient, highly computerized and automated means, and could result in the end of "the zombie sovereign power" and the formation of an "inevitably planetary society," distinguished by "a broad and deep commitment to public and private reason, including unfamiliar forms of sacrifice and behaviour change, a pragmatic vision for what is and is not 'essential', and a focusing of technical systems on equity and efficiency" (Bratton 2021: 1–4, 8–13, 19, 29–30). He presents a two-fold critique of negative biopolitics: having criticized negative biopolitics for being sceptical of biology and immediately associating any rehabilitation of the biological with a return to the promotion of eugenic ideas, Bratton blames negative biopolitics for interpreting the history of epidemiological interventions primarily as both a tool of coercive control and a hierarchical, normalizing discursive-technical apparatus, which equates all forms of statistical modelling and management of society to destructive surveillance (Bratton 2021: 3–4, 13–14, 37–38, 54–55, 127–128). However, one must admit that Bratton fails to avoid bias in his theory of planetary biopolitics.

Bratton postulates the necessity of planetary biopolitics and argues that the bio-governance of a post-pandemic world should be interested not only in ensuring the survival of life but also in its restoration, maintenance, and preservation. At the same time, Bratton urges us to consciously abandon illusions about our biological, epidemiological, and ecological condition, thereby advocating an inclusive, materialist, restorative, rationalist, and more demystified version of species-based post-pandemic biopolitics. Brattonian biopolitics accepts the evolutionary entanglement of mammals and viruses, the inseparability of death and life, and the responsibility of medicine to prevent unnecessary deaths by emphasizing that planetary thinking is incompatible with the conviction that the interconnectedness of populations and the struggle against contagion is an exceptional departure from the natural order, for an ethical, geo-historically realist planetarity starts with the realization that artificiality is by no means extraneous to human nature (Bratton 2021: 5, 120, 147–148). And while Bratton can't imagine post-pandemic politics without automation, he sees at least three fundamental changes needed to make automation applicable to planetary biopolitics. First, the fulfilment of basic living needs should be separated from the distortions of the social value of human beings resulting from hiring people to do menial jobs that otherwise would be performed by machines. Second, meeting basic living needs should also be separated from catastrophic ecological consequences. Third, automation should aim not only at the optimization of mechanisms but also at the liberation of public reason and collective intelligence (Bratton 2021: 89–90, 130). Finally, one cannot omit one more aspect of Bratton's positive biopolitics, one that is intertwined directly with planetary biopolitics, which the author calls *the ethics of being an object*. With this concept that echoes in Mbembe's formulation of the twofold process of the becoming-artificial of humanity and the becoming-human of objects and machines, Bratton advocates the need for a particular shift in ethics, a move to a position where the self and the body are conceived of as equal to objects, arguing that subjective intentionality loses its meaning when any individual – despite having the best of intentions – can unknowingly become a potential carrier of contagion, notwithstanding that phenomena of planetary nature, such as viruses or anthropogenic climate change, are indifferent to intentionality as such. Last but not least, Bratton observes that one of the main challenges the political philosophy is facing today is the need to conceptualize an ethics of being that would reconcile the extreme ethical subjectivism embodied in the popular slogan "Be the change you want to see in the world" and the implication of the privileged position of the subject in terms of establishing the material world (Bratton 2021: 105). One of Bratton's proposed solutions to this challenge is the expansion of the concept of bioethics to include not only the protection of individual privacy and the prevention of forced objectification but also a conscious ethical self-objectification whenever the need to care for other members of society for the sake of the common good arises (Bratton 2021: 103–106, 139–140). However, one is left with the impression that in establishing the ethics of being an object, Bratton does not perform any other intellectual manoeuvre except for taking one specific, even exceptional case – the outbreak of a pandemic – out of context and tries to define universal ethics accordingly, which does not make Bratton's theory of planetary biopolitics any more credible.

Despite being its avoidance, since Bratton himself, despite criticizing Agamben and Heidegger for their tendency to mystify this particular problem, treats reality as such an indisputable fact as the death itself (paradoxically, Bratton's book is titled *The Revenge of the Real*; in a certain sense, it can be said that even Bratton himself could not escape the revenge of the real). Second, when criticizing negative biopolitics taken as a whole, Bratton refers almost exclusively to Agamben, failing to cite any other theoretician more comprehensively. Moreover, Bratton's criticism of Agamben often teeters on the brink of an *ad hominem* attack, as in this case: "When a biopolitical philosophy was needed most, the author went mad" (Bratton 2021: 109). Third, for all of Bratton's criticism of right-wing populism, his vision of positive biopolitics virtually ignores social, racial, or any other inequality as if they do not exist, as it remains unclear how his proposed model of planetary biopolitics would ensure the rights of populations, traditionally considered the most vulnerable to the workings of biopower (ethnic, racial, sexual, and other minorities). Other authors also share similar reservations about Bratton's version of planetary biopolitics. Perhaps the most persuasive and detailed critique is presented by Peter Polack, an advocate of postcolonial computing, who has highlighted the inability of planetary-scale computation to consider the unpredictability of what he calls the *deep time of facts*, as each planetary fact always encounters heterogeneous cultural contexts, which in turn generate complex layers of new facts. Polack accuses Bratton of cultivating "false positivism," criticizes him for ignoring issues regarding privacy and individual agency in the name of a commitment to facts, and strongly disapproves of equating facticity to legality. Also, Polack fails to see why subjects should settle for the "ethics of being an object" and relinquish any decision-making over their inclusion in systems they don't have a say in developing, thereby highlighting the difference between data-driven inclusivity and inclusion in decision-making (Polack 2021). Finally, I would add that while seeing culture and politics as obstacles to viable planetary governance, as Bratton does, is one thing, the decision to abandon them altogether does not seem justified in any way.

4 Exploitative Geologies, New Temporalities: A Case for Geoplanetary Biopolitics?

To sum up these different and not necessarily inherently compatible theoretical perspectives, it can be argued that each of these four theorists – Yusoff, Chakrabarty, Mbembe, and Bratton – provides valuable insights that expand our understanding of the functioning of biopolitical mechanisms in the modern era and the impact of biopower on the planet's ecosystems. Yusoff's geological approach incorporates a highly material ecological dimension into biopolitics, linking biopolitics to exploitative practices of extraction through the interrelationship of geological and racial formations, thereby contesting the myth of Anthropocene neutrality and demonstrating the connections of race to the racialized extraction of non-human matter and the ensuing dehumanization of black subjects. Chakrabarty's dichotomy of global and planetary epistemes, in its turn, complements Yusoff's geological approach with a temporal dimension that establishes a nexus between human history and geological planetary time, thus emphasizing the need to recognize the role of humans as geophysical power and rethink the notion of biopolitics itself by including considerations that encompass not only population governance but also an injunction to respond to planetary-scale crises. Mbembe's neohumanist planetary biopolitics, based on the dialectic of exclusion and inclusion, helps to ground Chakrabarty's abstract and systemic notion of biopolitics, placing it in material contexts equally conditioned by the legacy of historical colonialism and contemporary racial and institutionalized violence. Finally, Bratton's planetary infrastructuralism, based on the ethics of being an object, though not sufficiently addressing contemporary practices of algorithmic discrimination and digital exclusion, allows us to understand the contribution of technological infrastructures and automation processes in shaping global biogovernance.

That said, none of these theoretical models seems in itself sufficient to adequately assess the role of race and racialization in contemporary biopolitics. Moreover, despite all technological advances, the fundamental question of biopolitics – who will be made to live and who will be allowed to die – remains closely intertwined with processes of racialization and extraction, ceaselessly operating on both global and planetary scales. Such a state of affairs, in turn, encourages one to formulate, at least in a very brief and concise way, some of the main principles of what could be called an integrated and multi-scale geoplanetary biopolitics that would overcome the aforementioned limitations of conventional biopolitics by encompassing the ecological and technological aspects of contemporary biogovernance and simultaneously recognizing the historical connections among colonialism, capitalism, and racialization. Unlike conventional biopolitical theories that have taken hold in scientific discourse, geoplanetary biopolitics emphasizes the need to reconsider the legacies of colonialism and imperialism, taking into account the material and affective – albeit not always explicit – influence of these historical formations on today's biogovernance regimes. Such geoplanetary biopolitics should be based on the idea of ecological justice and the assumption that biogovernance in the age of Anthropocene (or post-Anthropocene) should be concerned not only with hybrid governance of the biosphere and technosphere but would also provide certain safeguards that would prevent the distribution of racialized differential vulnerability, resulting in a disproportionate burden of global ecological transformations carried by racialized populations. In geoplanetary biopolitics, race should be conceptualized not only as a sociopolitical category but also as a process characterized by material connections with the geological formations of the planet. Such an updated notion of race, in turn, would allow us to connect the very origins of modern global infrastructures and planetary systems with the exploitative extraction-oriented practices of colonialism, industrial capitalism, and imperialism. Finally, such geoplanetary biopolitics would acknowledge that today's governance of life no longer aligns with national borders and operates on different scales simultaneously – local, national, global, and planetary. In this way, geoplanetary biopolitics would explain the interconnectedness of planetary processes, from ecological degradation to economic inequality, while highlighting the sustainability of the function of race as an axis of biopolitical control, which maintains its centrality in biopolitical calculations.

5 Conclusion

In terms of the big picture, it becomes evident that the possibilities for implementing planetary biopolitics in today's world are inseparable from the equal distribution of chances of liveability. After all, they ultimately depend not so much on the existing biopolitical frameworks as on their applicability in ensuring that the right to health is distributed to the world's populations equally and universally, which is not even worth discussing unless we find new ways to guarantee the survival of the world's populations in the aftermath of the COVID-19 and in the face of new emerging infectious diseases. The pandemic, however, has highlighted the symbiosis of human and non-human life on a planetary scale more than any other global historical event that preceded it.

While the perspectives on planetary biopolitics discussed in this chapter contrast sharply, they provide valuable insights into both the fundamental challenges the paradigm of planetary biopolitics is facing and the possible practical approaches to implementing it. The need to practice thinking in a truly planetary way also brings together postcolonial critique and the more conventional attempts at reformulating biopolitics. If we manage to expand the spatial dimension of biopolitics by discrediting the structural anthropocentric whiteness that is based on unequal power relations, replacing the Anthropocene with a new geology that gives credit to the workings of racialized assemblages, and come up with new ways of thinking that are not only global but also planetary, we could reconcile the vastness of the geobiological time with the highly affective structures of human historical time. While the works by the proponents of planetary biopolitics remain mostly flawed, most of them agree on the urgency to extend the right to life beyond the boundaries of the human world, thereby recognizing the ecological crisis and its threats on a planetary scale and the need to change the relationship with our surroundings, both close and planetary. And while the ethics of being an object may be seen as a threat to our highly valued individual subjectivity, it would not hurt to occasionally practice the ethics of being just one of many species if we are to secure truly universal, planetary conditions for life.

However, despite these valuable theoretical contributions, the prospects for equitable and realistic planetary biopolitics in a post-pandemic world remain highly uncertain. And while it is true that the newly proposed notion of geoplanetary biopolitics offers plenty of potential in reevaluating the material and affective legacies of colonialism and its highly racialized practices and some hope regarding the implementation of ecological justice, the balance that we must keep in recognizing the interconnectedness of all life forms on Earth, addressing global challenges, and maintaining respect for the agency and rights of individuals, communities and populations, crucial in the implementation of planetary biopolitics, remains nothing more than a meticulously crafted theoretical design, a posthumanist dream in wait for its implementation.

References

Anthias, Floya and Yuval-Davis, Nira. 1993. *Racialized Boundaries: Race, Nation, Gender, Colour and Class and the Anti-Racist Struggle*. London, New York: Routledge.

Bratton, Benjamin H. 2015. *The Stack: On Software and Sovereignty*. Cambridge, MA, London: MIT Press.

Bratton, Benjamin H. 2019. *The Terraforming*. Moscow: Strelka Press.

Bratton, Benjamin H. 2021. *The Revenge of the Real: Politics for a Post-pandemic World*. London, New York: Verso.

Butler, Judith and Athanasiou, Athena. 2013. *Dispossession: The Performative in the Political*. Cambridge, Malden: Polity Press.

Butler, Judith. 2022. *What World Is This? A Pandemic Phenomenology*. New York: Columbia University Press.

Chakrabarty, Dipesh. 2018. *The Crises of Civilization: Exploring Global and Planetary Histories*. Oxford: Oxford University Press.

Chakrabarty, Dipesh. 2021. *The Climate of History in a Planetary Age*. Chicago: The University of Chicago Press.

Chakrabarty, Dipesh. 2023a. "Foreword." In: *New Earth Histories: Geo-Cosmologies and the Making of the Modern World*. Chicago, London: University of Chicago Press.

Chakrabarty, Dipesh. 2023b. *One Planet, Many Worlds: The Climate Parallax*. Waltham, MA: Brandeis University Press.

Elias, Amy J. and Moraru, Christian (eds.). 2015. *The Planetary Turn: Relationality and Geoaesthetics in the Twenty-First Century*. Evanston: Northwestern University Press.

Fassin, Didier. 2018. *Life: A Critical User's Manual*. Cambridge: Polity Press.

Fields, Karen E. and Fields, Barbara J. 2012. *Racecraft: The Soul of Inequality in American Life*. London, New York: Verso.

Føllesdal, Dagfinn. 2009. "The *Lebenswelt* in Husserl." In: *Science and the Life-World: Essays on Husserl's Crisis of European Sciences*. David Hyder, Hans-Jörg Rheinberger (eds.). Stanford: Stanford University Press, 27–45.

Haff, Peter K. 2014. "Technology as a Geological Phenomenon: Implications for Human Well-Being." In: *A Stratigraphical Basis for the Anthropocene*, ed. C. N. Waters et al. (London: Geological Society, Special Publications), 301–309.

Hui, Yuk. 2020. "Philosophy and the Planetary." In: *Philosophy Today*, Volume 64, Issue 4 (Fall 2020): 865–869.

Jaspers, Karl. 2010. *Man in the Modern Age*. Oxon: Routledge.

Kovalyova, Natalia. 2022. "A Crisis to Think with: Mining the Biopolitics of COVID-19 in American Public Discourse." In: *Athena: filosofijos studijos*, 17: 123–140.

Latour, Bruno. 1993. *We Have Never Been Modern*. Harvard: Harvard University Press.

Loizidou, Elena. 2021. "Planetary Confinement: Bio-politics and Mutual Aid." In: *Law and Critique* 32: 133–138.

Malik, Kenan. 1996. *The Meaning of Race: Race, History and Culture in Western Society*. London: Macmillan Press.

Mbembe, Achille. 2017. *Critique of Black Reason*. Durham and London: Duke University Press.

Mbembe, Achille. 2019. *Necropolitics*. Durham and London: Duke University Press.

Mbembe, Achille. 2021a. "Futures of Life and Futures of Reason." In: *Public Culture*, 33 (1 (93)): 11–33.

Mbembe, Achille. 2021b. *Out of the Dark Night: Essays on Decolonization*. New York: Columbia University Press.

Mbembe, Achille. 2021c. "The Universal Right to Breathe." In: *Critical Inquiry*, 47 (S2): S58–S62.

Mbembe, Achille. 2024. *Brutalism*. Durham and London: Duke University Press.

Miles, Robert. 2000. "Apropos the Idea of Race… Again." In: *Theories of Race and Racism: A Reader*, eds. Back L., Solomos, J. London: Routledge, 125–143.

Miles, Robert and Brown, Malcolm. 2003. *Racism*. London, New York: Routledge.

Murji, Karim and Solomos, John (eds.). 2005. *Racialization: Studies in Theory and Practice*. Oxford: Oxford University Press.

Nasir, Muhammad A. 2016. "Biopolitics, Thanatopolitics and the Right to Life." In: *Theory, Culture and Society* 34 (1): 75–95.

Neyrat, Frédéric. 2016. "Planetary Antigones: The Environmental Situation and the Wandering Condition." In: *Qui Parle* 25 (1–2): 35–64.

Pele, Antonio and Riley, Stephen. 2025. "For a Right to Health Beyond Biopolitics: The Politics of Pandemic and the 'Politics of Life'." In: *Law, Culture and the Humanities* 21(1): 7–23.

Polack, Peter. 2021. "False Positivism: Why "Planetary Computation" and "Data-Driven Governance "Will Not Solve the World's Problems." In: *Real Life*, October 18th, 2021.

Povinelli, Elizabeth A. 2016. *Geontologies: A Requiem to Late Liberalism*. Durham, London: Duke University Press.

Rouvroy, Antoinette and Berns, Thomas. Trans. Libbrecht, E. 2013. "Algorithmic governmentality and prospects of emancipation: Disparateness as a precondition for individuation through relationships?" *Réseaux*, Vol. 177, No. 1, pp. 163–196, https://www.cairn-int.info/article-E_RES_177_0163--algorithmic-governmentality-and-prospect.htm. Accessed 4 September 2023.

Scheiner, Corinne. 2005. "Teleiopoiesis, Telepoesis, and the Practice of Comparative Literature." In: *Comparative Literature*, 57(3): 239–245.

Spivak, Gayatri Chakrabarty. 2003. *Death of a Discipline*. New York: Columbia University Press.

Stiegler, Bernard. 2016. *Automatic Society, Volume 1: The Future of Work*. Cambridge and Malden: Polity Press.

Stiegler, Bernard. 2018. *The Neganthropocene*. London: Open Humanities Press.

Tewari, Avantika. 2025. "Confronting Agamben on the Pandemic: Biopolitics, Class Struggle and Surveillance Capitalism." In: *Law, Culture and the Humanities* 21(1): 57–78.

Vatter, Miguel. 2022. "Planetary Health and the Biopolitics of Home." In: Lemm, V.; Vatter, M. (eds.) *The Viral Politics of Covid-19: Nature, Home, and Planetary Health.* Singapore: Springer Nature Singapore, 221–246.

Walton, Merrilyn. (ed.) 2019. *One Planet, One Health.* Sydney: University of Sydney Press.

Weinbaum, Alys E. 2019. *The Afterlife of Reproductive Slavery: Biocapitalism and Black Feminism's Philosophy of History.* Durham, London: Duke University Press.

Woodhouse, Edward J. 1988. "Planetary Governance and Biopolitics." In: *Politics and the Life Sciences*, 6(2): 240–241.

Yusoff, Kathryn. 2018. *A Billion Black Anthropocenes or None.* Minneapolis: University of Minnesota Press.

Yusoff, Kathryn. 2024. *Geologic Life: Inhuman Intimacies and the Geophysics of Race.* Durham, London: Duke University Press.

CHAPTER 8

Immunity and Symbiopolitics

Audronė Žukauskaitė

Abstract

The notion of immunity, as defined in biology in the middle of the twentieth century, draws a boundary between the "self" and the "nonself." In this respect, the notion of immunity is the perfect metaphor for biopolitical government: similar to the immune system, which fights everything that it sees as "nonself," biopolitical power discriminates against what it sees as "different" or "other." However, if we examine immunity not as a metaphor but as a phenomenon viewed from the perspective of contemporary biology, we have to admit that immunity comprises not only a defensive reaction towards an external, contagious element but also a positive reaction or so-called "tolerance." Thus, the defensive model of immunity should be complemented by a positive one, interpreting immunity as being entangled with its milieu. Alfred I. Tauber suggested that immunity should be seen as an ecological system that not simply reacts towards the external element but opens the negotiations between the "self" and "nonself" within the system. This model of ecological immunology is also a good methodological tool to rethink the notion of biopolitics: instead of seeing biopolitics as the opposition between a sovereign power and an oppressed individual, we can interpret it as a network of sympoietic interactions between individuals, technologies, and nonhuman others.

Keywords

immunity – immune system – autopoiesis – sympoiesis – biopolitics – community

1 Biopolitical Notion of Immunity

The notion of immunity has a long history in both medical and philosophical discourses. In philosophy, the notion of immunity was introduced by Donna J. Haraway, Jacques Derrida, Roberto Esposito, and other theorists. They all acknowledged the contradictory or aporetic nature of the term. Derrida mentions the notion of immunity in "Faith and Knowledge" (1998), *Rogues: Two*

 | DOI:10.1163/9789004748187_010

Essays on Reason (2005), and in his conversation with Giovanna Borradori (2003). For Derrida, the logic of immunity is always already trapped in the logic of autoimmunity: any democratic community that tries to protect itself from "foreign" elements (migrants, refugees, terrorists, etc.) risks destroying the essence of democracy and community; therefore it has to protect itself from this protection. In Derrida's words, "an autoimmunitary process is that strange behaviour where a living being, in a quasi-*suicidal* fashion, 'itself' works to destroy its own protection, to immunize itself *against* its 'own' immunity" (Derrida 2003: 94). In this sense, the immune system has to be directed towards the political body and work in an autoimmunitary regime to prevent its own destructive operationality. In Derrida's terminology, immunity is like a *pharmakon*, which means remedy and poison at the same time: "the *pharmakon* is another name, an old name, for this autoimmunitary logic" (Derrida 2003: 124). The *pharmakon* can protect the political body and keep it healthy and safe and simultaneously poison or destroy it. However, Derrida makes it clear that the paradox of (auto)immunity is not just a logical aporia or a kind of undecidability: this paradox is a necessary condition that not only allows an individual or collective body to protect its existence but also opens the possibility to meet the other: "autoimmunity is not an absolute ill or evil. It enables an exposure to the other, to *what* and to *who* comes – which means that it must remain incalculable. Without autoimmunity, with absolute immunity, nothing would ever happen or arrive: we would no longer wait, await, or expect, no longer expect one another, or expect any event" (Derrida 2005: 152). With absolute immunity, we would have a total closure that would prevent the advent of what is different or new.

The notion of immunity is also central in Roberto Esposito's works, where immunity is interpreted in biopolitical terms. For Esposito, the notion of immunity is always already a biopolitical term because it is etymologically associated with the notion of community: immunity and community derive from the Latin word "munus" which means "gift," "office," and "obligation" (Esposito 2011: 5–6; Esposito 2010: 1–12). Thus, immunity would imply the exemption from the condition of gift-giving, whereas community is based precisely on this obligation. In this respect, community is always struggling to keep its boundaries and protect itself from "others." On the other hand, without these "others," community would lose its meaning. Esposito is trying to solve this aporia by pointing out that the immune system has two functions: besides the defensive or reactionary aspects of the immune system, we can see the positive functioning of immunity (so-called "immune tolerance"). "What we want to draw attention to is how this leads to the reversal of a common perception: it is not autoimmunity, with all its lethal consequences, including death, that requires explanation, but rather its absence" (Esposito 2011: 164). Esposito thinks that the positive functioning of immunity (so-called "immune tolerance") can be translated into social and political terms and establish a new model of community. In the final chapter of *Immunitas*, called "Common immunity," Esposito refers to more recent research in immunology, which reconsiders immunity as an ecosystem that constantly evolves, changes, and moves the boundary between the "self" and "nonself." Esposito implies that this double function of immunity can be transposed into the field of biopolitics – instead of focusing on the negative functions of biopolitics, we should move towards positive or affirmative biopolitics.

However, it seems that Esposito's project of affirmative biopolitics gets trapped in the aporias of negative dialectics. Even if *Immunitas* ends with a promise of new forms of co-immunity, Esposito's other books, such as *Communitas* or *Terms of the Political*, do not give a single clear idea about what constitutes this new community. Esposito relies on negative definitions of community, defining it not as a place of identity, belonging, and appropriation but, on the contrary, a place of plurality, difference, and alterity (Esposito 2013: 55). In other words, when we try to grasp what it means to be in a community in Esposito's terms, it seems that this can be expressed only in negative terms. Inspired by Maurice Blanchot and Jean-Luc Nancy, Esposito describes community in terms of absence or deprivation: "If the community always consists of others and never of itself, this suggests that its presence is constitutively inhabited by an absence of subjectivity, of identity, of property. [...] [T]he being of community is the interval of difference, the spacing that brings us into relation with others in a common non-belonging, in this loss of what is proper that never adds up to a common 'good'. Common is only lack and not possession, property, or appropriation" (Esposito 2010: 138–9).

Esposito's latest book, *Common Immunity* (2023), examines the recent COVID-19 pandemic and the urgent need to create "herd immunity," which should work not only in a particular community but also on a planetary scale. However, according to Esposito, even in this unique situation, we can discern the same negative dialectics, which reintroduces the relationship between immunity and privilege and allows the old immunitary dispositifs to re-emerge in ever-new forms. On the one hand, common immunity looks like a unique chance to create a global community; on the other hand, once the vaccine was produced, this eventual community was fractured by many lines of separation and biopolitical dispositifs. Again, the newly developed vaccine works as an ambivalent *pharmakon* because "the instrument that was potentially designed to reduce inequalities through global immunization now risks multiplying them, reproducing immunization's initially divisive and exclusionary character. Far from coinciding with *communitas, immunitas* is detaching itself from it again, regressing toward its original meaning of privilege" (Esposito 2023: 189). It seems that Esposito cannot overcome his negative predisposition and is unable to formulate immunity in positive terms.

For this reason, I would like to return to Derrida's take on (auto)immunity, even if Esposito underestimates it as supposedly lacking a communitarian dimension. As Esposito formulates it, "certain relevant differences remain vis-à-vis the formation of the category of immunity that in Derrida emerge as somewhat extemporaneous, in a sense that immunity is linked neither with the theme of community (which Derrida rejects in favour of the weaker concept, from my point of view, of friendship) nor with that of biopolitics, which is utterly extraneous to his thought" (Esposito, Paparcone 2006: 53). However, I would argue that Derrida's take on immunity and community operates in a different logic, which is aporetic but – at the same time – creative and productive. In *Rogues*, Derrida asserts that community as co-immunity necessarily implies the logic of *différance*, which means difference and delay at the same time: "The formalization of this autoimmune law was there carried out around the *community as auto-co-immunity* (the common of community having in common the same duty or charge [*munus*] as the immune, as well as the auto-co-immunity of humanity [...]" (Derrida 2005: 35). According to Derrida, democracy is defined by the lack of "the proper and the selfsame," in other words, "the autoimmune process we have been analyzing within democracy consists always in a renvoi, a referral or deferral, a sending or putting off" (Derrida 2005: 35). The autoimmune logic requires that democracy never coincides with itself and is always sent off elsewhere or put off until better times (these are two meanings of the French word *renvoyer*). In this respect, even without mentioning biopolitics, Derrida formulates a very important problem: how can anything (a biological or political body) exist without a proper meaning? How can anything exist while being constantly replaced or delayed? This is the problem that appears at the centre of the theory of autopoiesis: to remain what it is, a body (a molecule, an individual, or a community) has to be closed, immunize itself from the outside, and have a boundary; however, to maintain its existence, to change and evolve, it has to be open to the environment. In Derrida's terms, this is the problem not only of *pharmakon* but also of *différance*: how to be inside and outside at the same time? How can we define the contagious other if we cannot define the proper self?

2 Biological Notion of Immunity

To answer these questions, we should take a closer look into how the notion of "self" is formulated in the history of immunology. From its formulation in the middle of the twentieth century, the immune system was defined around the notions of "self" and "nonself": the immune system ignores the "self" and fights against the "nonself" or "other." However, the distinction between the "self" and the "nonself" is not so clear if we want to explain it biologically. What remains to be explained is what defines this "self" and why the immune system is silent in relation to its own cells and tissues. What happens when a part of the so-called "self" changes and becomes a stranger to itself? Is the biological "self" identical to the philosophical and psychological notions of individuality? As Alfred I. Tauber explains, the notion of selfhood was not only imported from philosophical discourse but also quickly became an idiom, which was explained as if it grew within the science of immunology (Tauber 2017: 42). The notion of the "self," which comprises both the organismal self and the immunological self, was a very convenient and recognizable model to think about our immunological identity. However, as immunology developed, some important questions had to be answered. It is obvious that the immunological "self" is never given all at once but develops throughout the organism's life. This "self" becomes even more blurry if we take into account the discovery of induced immunity, which means that immunity can be manipulated artificially. Another important observation is that the immune system has more than one response – in its exchange with the environment, the organism normally reacts not in a defensive but in an assimilative manner (eating and breathing). The immunological "self" can also be nonreactive or silent in relation to the cells of other organisms, such as in the case of pregnancy. There is clear evidence that, long after delivery, foetal cells are found in maternal bodies, creating a case of microchimerism. Why does the immune system not attack these cells? And, on the contrary, why does the immune system *react* to the cells of the same organism in the case of autoimmune diseases? Why does the immune system treat the "self" as if it is the "other"?

All these questions signal that the notion of immunity is a complex concept, and its reconceptualization is also changing. As Tauber argues, rather than being understood as a defensive reaction towards an external, contagious element, immunity is now conceived as a network that keeps the balance in the organismal "self." In other words, it is not a negative reaction towards a foreign element but a normal functioning that needs to be explained. As Tauber points out, "When immune reactions are conceived in terms of normal physiology and open exchange with the environment, where borders dividing host and foreign are elusive and changing, host defence is only part of the immune system's functions, which actually comprise two basic tasks: to preserve host *integrity* (protection) and to establish organismic *identity*" (Tauber 2017: 117). In other words, immunity should be examined not in its negative and reactive state (as defence), but in its positive state (as "tolerance" or immune silence). Examined from this perspective, immunity is explained not in terms of an opposition between "self" and "nonself" but as a self-referential system.

This conceptual shift can be related to the work of immunologist Niels Jerne and his "network theory," which explains immunity as a self-referential system. It is interesting that Donna J. Haraway also points out the importance of Jerne's idea that the immune system has to be understood not as a protection of the individual "self" but as a changing network based on self-regulation and self-organization. "Jerne's basic idea was that any antibody molecule must be able to act functionally as both antibody to some antigen *and* as antigen for the production of an antibody to itself, albeit at another region of 'itself'" (Haraway 2013: 291). In this sense, the immune system is understood as a network capable of recognizing and mirroring the antigen in such a way that there is nothing external that the immune system has not already mirrored internally. "'Self' and 'other' lose their rationalistic oppositional quality and become subtle plays of partially mirrored readings and responses. The notion of the *internal image* is the key to the theory, and it entails the premise that every member of the immune system is capable of interacting with every other member" (Haraway 2013: 291). Thus, the immune system is understood as an internal network that reacts not to an external "invader" but to its internal structuring.

Tauber also examines Jerne's network theory as a major shift in immunity theorizing. As Tauber explains, Jerne proposed the idea that the immune system is made of interlocking recognizing units so that each component reacts with the other within the system, and, in this way, they all together form a self-referential network. In this model, the antibody has two roles: active and passive: "So in addition to the active binding of antigen, Jerne suggested that antibody could also act as the target of another antibody by presenting itself as an antigen through its so-called *idiotypic* domains. On this view, immunoglobulin behaves as both antibody (as originally regarded) and antigen to a corresponding antibody that reacts with its unique *idiotope*" (Tauber 2017: 60). The immune system reacts to the external antigens only to the extent that these elements are recognized in the internal "library" of antibodies. "In other words, Jerne postulated that the amino acid sequences of immunoglobulins share structural homologies with all antigens to which the organism might respond – that is, 'internal images' represent that external universe" (Tauber 2017: 60).

Thus, the immune system performs a dialogue between antibodies, which play two roles: either of the "recognizer" or the "recognized." Neither the "recognizer" nor the "recognized" have any essential characteristics of "self" or "nonself." Rather they are, in Derrida's terms, signifiers referring to other signifiers, and in this sense, immunity can be understood as a self-referential structure of language. The "other" is something that simply disturbs that structure and activates a response.

The immune system, seen from this perspective, cannot be explained by the "self" and "nonself" distinction because, strictly speaking, the immune network can recognize only itself. Every element is always already within the system, and what is external or "other" is either invisible or appears as "nonsense." The distinction between "self" and "other" can be conceptualized only from the observer's point of view, whereas the immune network is always immanent to itself and cannot reflect its outside. As Tauber points out, "Jerne's network conception [was] built on *self-recognition*, which then reconfigured 'autoimmunity' (self-recognition) from aberrancy to the normative organizational rule of immune function" (Tauber 2017: 62). Immune tolerance or silence does not need a specific explanation because the immune system knows only itself. The originality of Jerne's model lies in the fact that it denies the subject-object structure, which implies the observer's perspective and suggests that immunity is an immanent structure based on self-survey. As Tauber observes, "Jerne's innovation offered a model of immune function independent of agency, and with that move, he highlighted the difference between the observer's perspective and the network's" (Tauber 2017: 65). Thus, for Jerne, immune network perceives and observes itself in self-referential loops, which can be discussed in terms of autopoietic systems.

The notion of autopoiesis was introduced in Humberto Maturana and Francisco Varela's *Autopoiesis and Cognition* (1980). A simple example of an autopoietic system is a unicellular organism that is capable of maintaining and recreating its organization despite multiple chemical reactions taking place in it. Thus, the main characteristic of an autopoietic system is its self-organization, self-maintenance, and its constant self-reproduction within a boundary. However, a living being cannot survive without energy and nutrients, and, for this reason, it is connected to the environment. The environment triggers an autopoietic system and engenders some changes within its structure. However, even after undergoing some structural changes, the model of the organization of the system does not change. Therefore, autopoietic entities are said to be *closed* on the level of organization but *open* on the level of structure. As Evan Thompson points out, "The self-transcending movement of life is none other than metabolism, and metabolism is none other than the biochemical instantiation of the autopoietic organization. That organization must remain invariant – otherwise, the organism dies – but the only way autopoiesis can stay in place is through the incessant material flux of metabolism. In other words, the operational *closure* of autopoiesis demands that the organism be an *open system*" (Thompson 2009: 85). In other words, to stay alive, a system has to communicate with the environment and change because a total closure would mean death.

Varela was trying to theorize immunity as an autopoietic system and reconcile his theory with Jerne's network hypothesis. In "Immu-knowledge: The Process of Somatic Individuation," Varela and Anspach argue that one must "drop the notion of the immune system as a defensive device built to address external events" and instead "conceive it in terms of self-assertion, establishing a molecular identity by the maintenance of circulation levels of molecules through the entire distributed network [...]. This idea is strictly parallel to the species network giving an ecosystem an identity within an environment" (Varela, Anspach 1991: 78–79). In other words, Varela and Anspach analyse an immune system as a self-referential autopoietic system operating through recurrent causality. In this respect, the immune system expresses a certain kind of knowledge, or cognition, and is processing information that is necessary to maintain the organism's integrity and identity: "We argue that the immune system is a cognitive network, not only because of properties which it shares with the brain, but also, more interestingly, because in both cases we have similar (or at least comparable) global properties of biological networks giving rise to cognitive behaviour as emergent properties" (Varela, Anspach 1991: 70). The immune system is understood as an autopoietic cognitive network, which can easily connect to other autopoietic networks of different complexity.

In this respect, the immune system is seen as a part of more general ecological networking. Varela and Anspach go so far as to draw a comparison between an immune system and a planetary system: "Let us transpose the metaphor to immunobiology, and suggest that the body is like Earth, a textured environment for diverse and highly interactive populations of individuals. The individuals in this case are the white blood cells or lymphocytes which constitute the immune system" (Varela, Anspach 1991: 69). The lymphocytes generate different molecular populations within the body, similar to living species which generate diversity within an ecosystem. The immune system is like "a microcosmic version of Gaia" (Varela, Anspach 1991: 69), which can maintain its balance through self-referential processes. However, what remains problematic in this autopoietic approach is how to define the other. If the cognitive network only knows itself, how can it communicate with other organisms and other ecosystems? As Tauber explains, in this theory, the "nonself" appears only as a perturbation or as informational noise: "Simply, the *other* [nonself] does not exist in this closed system as Jerne originally proposed. [...] ANT [Autonomous Network Theory], locked into seeing only itself and blind to the *other*, fails to define the other as other, which then can only be identified as 'foreign' from an exterior point of view [...]" (Tauber 2017: 237). In other words, if the immune system knows only itself, how can it coexist with other systems, and, in general, how does it recognize the "nonself"?

Cary Wolfe gives a Derridean answer to this question: "the autopoietic closure of the system – whether social or psychic – is precisely what *connects* it to its environment" (Wolfe 2010: 257). Wolfe refers to Niklas Luhmann's explanation that "[t]he concept of a self-referentially closed system does not contradict the system's *openness to the environment*. Instead, in the self-referential mode of operation, closure is a form of broadening possible environmental contacts; closure increases, by constituting elements more capable of being determined, the complexity of the environment that is possible for the system" (Luhmann 1995: 37). In other words, autopoietic self-reference does not imply solipsistic closure; on the contrary, the more autopoietic the system is, the more complex it is; and the more complex the system is, the more sensitive or conscious of its environment it is. Wolfe argues that we should reconsider the principle of "openness from closure" (Wolfe 2020: 142) as the main characteristic of second-order systems. The system is open from closure in the sense that it interiorizes an exterior heterogeneous element into the very system, thus forming a new re-entry, a new loop. Autopoietic referentiality is not only the "repetition of the same" but also the inclusion and repetition of contingent elements that are integrated into that system. And the more the system can integrate contingency, the more successful and adaptable it is. As Luhmann points out, "In systems that are successful in evolutionary terms, more independence typically amounts to a greater dependency on the environment [...]. But all of this can happen only on the basis of the system's operative closure" (Luhmann 2000: 158, cited in Wolfe 2010: 222). Now, to translate it into terms of the immune system, we can say that successful immunity amounts to a greater dependency on the environment and the capacity to introduce a contingent element within that system.

3 Sympoietic Biopolitics

Thus, can we reframe the question of immunity in ecological terms so that immunity refers not to the defensive reaction of an insular organism but to the interrelations between different organisms or individuals? And if yes, can we avoid a contradiction between the so-called closure of autopoietic systems and the openness of ecological or communal beings? As Tauber argues, ecological immunology does not simply mean that every individual is in a relationship with the environment, which is self-obvious. It means that every individual is in a relationship with its internal ecosystem and external ecosystem. Every individual is a holobiont, composed of its internal microbiome and the resident symbionts living in the gut, skin, and on other surfaces. This internal ecology is responsible not only for normal physiology but also for the functioning of the immune system: "an individual's immune system itself is in part created by the resident microbiome, the consortium of microbes that live in commensal association with the resident animal constituents" (Tauber 2022: 142). In this sense, the opposition between the "self" and the "other" should be replaced by the multiple interactions between the internal ecosystem (a holobiont) and the external ecosystem (the environment). It is important to point out that these interrelations evolve and change during the entire life span of the organism, modifying both the internal holobiont and the external environment.

The idea that the "self" is a holobiont composed of a host and several symbionts is not new to developmental biologists. Examining an organism according to anatomical, developmental, physiological, genetic, and immunological criteria, they argue that "we have never been individuals" because all organisms are related to each other in an all-pervading symbiosis (Gilbert et al. 2012). However, the notion of holobiont changes not only our understanding of the animal world but also the idea of what it means to be human. In a more recent article, Gilbert observes that "The holobiont is powerful, in part, because it is not limited to nonhuman organisms. It also changes what it means to be a person" (Gilbert 2017: 75). Recent research in immunology reveals that there is no such thing as an individual "self" because our bodies couldn't survive without hosting microbial organisms. This means that symbiosis is not an exceptional or marginal case but a fundamental principle of life. "These major symbiotic webs rule the planet, and within these big symbioses are the smaller symbiotic webs of things we call organisms. [...] Symbiosis is the way of life on earth; we are all holobionts by birth" (Gilbert 2017: 84). But if we all are holobionts by birth, what do these modes of symbiosis and co-immunity mean for us and other species? Are we ready to give up the philosophical and psychological notion of the individual "self"?

However, philosophy has already offered many models to think of the individual "self" in terms of ecological multiplicity. Gilles Deleuze and Félix Guattari made many attempts to disarticulate the idea of an organism and open it to becoming and "unnatural participations." For them, an organism is an assemblage-like construction, the body without organs, which demonstrates the disorganization of the organism and the denaturalization of nature. Deleuze and Guattari are interested in different modes of becoming, which are defined as expansion, propagation, occupation, contagion, and peopling. These becomings are organized around two types of multiplicities: one is organized by descent, filiation, or heredity (that is, internal self-organization), and the other – by co-functioning of heterogeneous elements found in symbiosis and a holobiont. "We oppose epidemic to filiation, contagion to heredity, peopling by contagion to sexual reproduction, sexual production. Bands, human or animal, proliferate by contagion, epidemics, battlefields, and catastrophes. [...] Unnatural participations or nuptials are the true Nature spanning the kingdoms of nature" (Deleuze, Guattari 2004: 266). Filiation or heredity connects more or less homogeneous beings, while symbiosis or contagion occurs between entirely heterogeneous beings: it can be a human being, an animal, a bacterium, a virus, or a molecule. Heterogeneous becomings imply a multiplicity, which, in turn, implies symbiosis: "Each multiplicity is symbiotic; its becoming ties together animals, plants, microorganisms, mad particles, a whole galaxy" (Deleuze, Guattari 2004: 275). However, it is important to ask whether every symbiosis is profitable, increasing the partner's vital potential, or is it lethally dangerous, as in the case of contagion.

Haraway also insists on the contingent and undetermined mode of every multiplicity. However, she stresses symbiotic cooperation and sympoietic entanglements. The distinction between internal multiplicities and external multiplicities here is discussed as the dialectics between autopoiesis and sympoiesis: autopoietic systems are seen as homeostatic, predictable, and development-oriented, whereas sympoietic systems are seen as allopoietic (producing otherness), unpredictable, and evolutionary oriented. Sympoietic systems, which also include autopoietic systems as their components, can maintain their identity and the status quo and, at the same time, have the potential to change and adapt to changes coming from the environment. And yet, Haraway admits that the opposition between autopoiesis and sympoiesis is a false one: "As long as autopoiesis does not mean self-sufficient 'self-making,' autopoiesis and sympoiesis, foregrounding and backgrounding different aspects of systemic complexity, are in generative friction, or generative enfolding, rather than opposition" (Haraway 2016: 61). According to Haraway, autopoiesis can explain the internal complexity of individuals, whereas sympoiesis is a better term to explain the collaborative assemblages which acquire their identity in the process of interaction and becoming. By fusing different components, sympoiesis creates more complex life forms and gives rise to new emergent properties.

Haraway refers to Margulis's notion of the holobiont, which indicates an organism plus persisting symbionts, such as the poster critter *Mixotricha paradoxa* (Margulis, Sagan 2001). For Haraway, the notion of holobiont questions the idea of a self-organized individual and indicates that all living beings appear as a result of dynamic organizing processes. In this respect, Haraway thinks that sympoiesis "is a word proper to complex, dynamic, responsive, situated, historical systems. [...] Sympoiesis enfolds autopoiesis and generatively unfurls and extends it" (Haraway 2016: 58). And yet, Haraway takes the notion of holobiont even further by trying to decentralize the relationships between a host and its symbionts: "my use of *holobiont* does not designate host + symbionts because all of the players are symbionts to each other, in diverse kinds of relationalities and with varying degrees of openness to attachments and assemblages with other holobionts" (Hawaway 2016: 60). The idea that "all of the players are symbionts to each other" echoes Bruno Latour's formulation that every agent is trying to manipulate another in such a way that all borders between an organism and its environment, between the inside and the outside are subverted. "Since all living agents follow their own intentions all along, modifying their neighbors as much as possible, there is no way to distinguish between the environment to which the organism is adapting and the point at which its own action begins" (Latour 2017: 100). However, this subversion poses another methodological question: if the borders (and all individual boundaries) are subverted, how can we eventually distinguish between organisms and their environments?

The subversion of borders opens the possibility to think about planetary symbiopolitics, which connects all human and nonhuman agents in the "waves of actions," which are not necessarily purposeful but might be contingent and unintentional. The recent COVID-19 pandemic is a good example illustrating that biopolitics is now operating on a planetary scale incorporating both human and nonhuman agents, which are holobionts to each other. It means that the relationships between them cannot be explained in terms of causality or intentional calculations. Their co-functioning, or sympoiesis, is unpredictable and contingent: in some cases, it creates conditions for better liveability, whereas in others, it fosters conditions of a lethal contagion. As Latour points out, "it is miscalculations that end up creating, randomly and without the slightest hint of a providence, conditions of liveability that other living things, downstream, have seized on, the way the famous oxygen-producing bacteria have, unintentionally, enabled other organisms to try new solutions; or the way deforestation in southern China opened up 'great opportunities,' as we know, for COVID-19" (Latour 2021a: 66). Similar to oxygen-producing bacteria, which, unintentionally, invented new conditions for living, human agents invented conditions for a pandemic to appear.

This is a clear sign that every biopolitics is always already symbiopolitics, affecting the conditions of liveability of both human and nonhuman symbionts. As Latour points out, the ecological crisis makes us reassess the notion of the human: "In the health crisis, it may be true that humans as a whole are fighting against viruses, even if they have no interest in us and go their way from throat to throat, killing us without meaning to. The situation is tragically reversed in the ecological change; this time, the pathogen whose terrible virulence has changed the living conditions of all the inhabitants of the planet is not the virus at all – it is humanity!" (Latour 2021b). The anthropomorphic mode of biopolitics, where humans manipulate everything around them, is now replaced by the nonhuman symbiopolitics, where humans circulate alongside other pathogens. The model of symbiopolitics makes the question of community irrelevant since every individual is always already a community, composed both of an internal ecosystem and an external ecosystem, co-functioning with human and nonhuman others. Latour makes it clear that the classical definition of community and society – presuming humans among themselves – makes no sense because humans are interrelated with nonhuman and inhuman others in sympoietic assemblages of different scales. In this respect, affirmative biopolitics should not be invented (as it already exists) but discerned and conceptualized in terms of multiplicity (Deleuze and Guattari), sympoiesis (Haraway), and agency (Latour). Such an affirmative model of symbiopolitics reframes the opposition between immunity and community: to acquire immunity, I do not have to protect the "self" from "nonself" or "other"; on the contrary, the "other" is what makes "my" immunity possible. In this model, the differences and heterogeneities are not rejected or suppressed but affirmatively transformed so that they produce a sympoiesis of a different kind. It reminds us that symbiopolitics requires us to prioritize those philosophical models that can affirmatively conceptualize differences and heterogeneities.

References

Deleuze, G., Guattari, F. 2004. *A Thousand Plateaus*: *Capitalism and Schizophrenia*, translated by B. Massumi. London, New York: Continuum.

Derrida, J. 1998. "Faith and Knowledge: The Two Sources of 'Religion' at the Limits of Reason Alone", in *Religion*, edited by J. Derrida, G. Vattimo, trans. D. Webb et al., 1–79.

Derrida, J. 2003. "Autoimmunity: Real and Symbolic Suicides: A Dialogue with Jacques Derrida", Trans Pascale-Anne Brault and Michael Naas. In: *Philosophy in a Time of Terror: Dialogues with Jürgen Habermas and Jacques Derrida*, edited by G. Borradori. Chicago: The University of Chicago Press, 85–136.

Derrida, J. 2005. *Rogues: Two Essays on Reason*, translated by Pascale-Anne Brault and Michael Naas. Stanford: Stanford University Press.

Esposito, R.; Paparcone, A. 2006. "Interview: Roberto Esposito", *Diacritics* 36 (2): 49–56, https://doi.org/10.1353/dia.2008.0010. Accessed 7 February 2024.

Esposito, R. 2010. *Communitas: The Origin and Destiny of Community*, translated by T. Campbell. Stanford: Stanford University Press.

Esposito, R. 2011. *Immunitas: The Protection and Negation of Life*, translated by Z. Hanafi. Cambridge: Polity Press.

Esposito, R. 2013. *Terms of the Political: Community, Immunity, Biopolitics*, translated by R. N. Welch. New York: Fordham University Press.

Esposito, R. 2023. *Common Immunity: Biopolitics in the Age of the Pandemic*, translated by Zakiya Hanafi, Cambridge: Polity Press.

Gilbert, S. F., Sapp, J., Tauber, A. I. 2012. "A Symbiotic View of Life: We Have Never Been Individuals," *The Quarterly Review of Biology* 87 (4): 325–341, https://doi.org/10.1086/668166. Accessed 7 February 2024.

Gilbert, S. F. 2017. "Holobiont by Birth: Multilineage Individuals as the Concretion of Cooperative Processes", *Arts of Living on a Damaged Planet*, edited by A. Tsing, H. Swanson, E. Gan and N. Bubandt, Minneapolis: University of Minnesota Press, 73–89.

Haraway, D. J. 2013 [1989]. "The Biopolitics of Postmodern Bodies: Constitutions of Self in Immune System Discourse", in *Biopolitics: A Reader*, edited by T. Campbell and A. Sitze. Durham and London: Duke University Press, 274–309.

Haraway, D. J. 2016. *Staying with the Trouble: Making Kin in the Chthulucene*. Durham, London: Duke University Press.

Latour, B. 2017. *Facing Gaia: Eighth Lectures on the New Climatic Regime*, translated by Catherine Porter. Cambridge: Polity Press.

Latour, B. 2021a. *After Lockdown. A Metamorphosis*, translated by J. Rose. Cambridge: Polity Press.

Latour, B. 2021b. "Is This a Dress Rehearsal?", *Critical Inquiry*, 47: S2.

Luhmann, N. 1995. *Social Systems*, translated by J. Bednarz, Jr. with D. Baecker. Stanford: Stanford University Press.

Luhmann, N. 2000. *Art as Social System*, translated by E. M. Knodt. Stanford: Stanford University Press.

Margulis, L., Sagan, D. 2001. "The Beast with Five Genomes", *Natural History*, 110 (5): 38–41.

Maturana, H., Varela, F. 1980. *Autopoiesis and Cognition: The Realization of the Living.* Dordrecht, Boston, London: Reidel Publishing Company.

Tauber, A. I. 2018. *Immunity: The Evolution of an Idea.* Oxford: Oxford University Press.

Tauber, A. I. 2022. *The Triumph of Uncertainty: Science and Self in the Postmodern Age.* Budapest, Vienna, New York: CEU Press.

Thompson, E. 2009. "Life and Mind: from Autopoiesis to Neurophenomenology", in Bruce Clarke and Mark B. N. Hansen (eds.). *Emergence and Embodiment: New Essays on Second-Order Systems Theory.* Durham and London: Duke University Press, 77–93.

Varela, F., Anspach, M. 1991. "Immu-Knowledge: the Process of Somatic Individuation", in William Irvin Thompson (ed), *Gaia 2 – Emergence: The New Science of Becoming.* Hudson: Lindisfarne Press, 68–85.

Wolfe, C. 2010. *What Is Posthumanism?* Minneapolis: University of Minnesota Press.

Wolfe, C. 2020. "What 'the Animal' Can Teach 'the Anthropocene", *Angelaki,* 25:3, 131–145, https://doi.org/10.1080/0969725X.2020.1754033. Accessed 7 February 2024.

Conclusions: Toward a Planetary Biopolitics

J. D. Mininger, Denis Petrina, Aistis Žekevičius and Audronė Žukauskaitė

The monograph offers a twofold perspective on the notion of biopolitics: on the one hand, it examines the negative effects of the pandemic, which made the implicit social, racial, and geopolitical inequalities explicit; on the other hand, it has made evident the need to reformulate biopolitics, and governmentality, in positive terms so that it would be capable of operating on the planetary scale.

The first part of the book examines the negative effects of biopolitics. In the article "Philosophy as Immunity and Contagion," J. D. Mininger expresses severe doubts over the effectiveness of philosophical inquiry as an immunization against false discourse and prejudice since seeking truth through philosophical inquiry may not necessarily lead to genuine self-awareness or a risk-taking process of self-inquiry that challenges existing beliefs and assumptions. Deploying Karl Jaspers' concept of a "limit situation" to consider these matters and analyzing Plato's famous account of the death of Socrates as a foundational historical and conceptual moment for philosophy, the author problematizes the metaphor of philosophy as an inoculation against false discourse further by suggesting that philosophy should be first and foremost concerned not about finding solace in the face of suffering but about engaging in rigorous truth-seeking even in the most challenging circumstances. By reminding the reader(s) that the task of philosophy lies in the pursuit of truth rather than the possession of it, J. D. Mininger seemingly comes to terms with the idea that truth always remains just out of reach since philosophy itself embodies an "essential position of otherness," as Foucault would have it, and requires a willingness to embrace uncertainty and ambiguity in the time marked by limit(ing) and liminal shifts.

Denis Petrina's chapter "Total Lockdown: the Pandemic and Affective Disorders" develops a critical account of biopower as exercised through the management of the pandemic. At its core is the triad of security, order, and care – a *dispositif* whose apparent benevolence also served as a "smokescreen" behind which a profound structural insensitivity to affective life was concealed. Referring to Foucault's work on discourse and Arthur's concept of the sanitizing force, the chapter shows how pandemic governance operated through a logic of the so-called *discursive sanitization*: the reduction of lived, singular experiences of grief, fear, anxiety, and depression to quantifiable,

 | DOI:10.1163/9789004748187_011

medically codified symptoms within a hegemonic regime of truth. This regime, though expressed statistically, does not merely represent reality but produces it as well, all the while obscuring the rich heterogeneity of affective experience beneath a veil of normative, statistical monumentality.

"Total Lockdown," as conceptualized in the chapter, therefore refers not only to a *political imposition* driven by neoliberal governmentality (whose relation to biopolitics is also examined) but also to an *ontological condition*: the reduction of *vita activa* – life in its affirmative, unfolding potentiality – to a state of cold, indifferent suspension. Within this suspension, the biopolitical insistence on security encounters its dark double – existential insecurity – generated largely by what Grossberg calls "the affective epidemic": the strategic deployment of fear and stress to consolidate the *status quo*. The state's response – cloaked in the rhetoric of security and care – is further problematized through Prozorov's notion of biopower as *unrequited love*: vertical, asymmetrical, and, ultimately, caring about the subject only insofar as it ensures the welfare of the population as a whole.

This configuration resonates with the logic and pragmatics of negative biopolitics, wherein governance reduces life to bare survival, flattening rather than enabling the transformative capacities of affect. Engaging the Deleuzian concept of *sad passions*, inherited from Spinoza, the chapter identifies depression as a complex constellation where the medical, personal, and sociopolitical converge, signalling a profound failure to care. Referring to thinkers from affect theory who have addressed the perennial challenge of sad passions both within or beyond the pandemic context, the chapter ultimately proposes a shift from *structured feelings* toward infrastructures of feeling – infra-level forms of resistance, gestures, and micro-practices that, on the one hand, immanently defy the hegemonic discourse, and, on the other, reconfigure our relation to care, solidarity, and shared vulnerability.

The COVID-19 pandemic exposed not only the biopolitical governance of life but also the existing structural racial inequality on a planetary scale, allowing us to see the racialized workings of biopolitical mechanisms that differentiate which lives are deemed valuable and thus worthy of living and which are regarded as mere commodities with an implicit expiry date. Instead of being celebrated as a rare opportunity to redefine our relationship with fragile ecosystems of the planet, critically reevaluate the extractive nature of late capitalism, and seek ways to recognize the mutual vulnerability of all forms of life and foster solidarity, the pandemic has merely acted as a magnifying glass, reflecting the full extent of uneven distribution of structural inequalities, if not further entrenching and intensifying the racialized necropolitical regimes of extraction and exclusion.

Aistis Žekevičius' chapter "Pandemic and Race: Un(fore)seen Circumstances, Same Old Biopolitics?" demonstrates that race has long served as a tool for biopolitical categorization, allowing one to decide on who is deemed useful and who is considered disposable, and the COVID-19 pandemic has demonstrated how racial capitalism structures global health responses, relegating marginalized populations to the status of expendable resources. Applied to pandemic conditions, Sara Ahmed's notion of use allows us to see how the ability to avoid direct exposure to the virus became a privilege, delineated along racial lines throughout the pandemic. The neoliberal economic framework only reinforces this highly racialized dynamic through concepts such as Gary Becker's "statistical value of life," introducing the economic dimension into pandemic biopolitics, where the chances of survival are translated into economic calculations that ultimately prioritize some lives over others. Finally, the work of Eugene T. Richardson and Alexandre White situates the spheres of public health, epidemiology, and infectious disease control within a (post)colonial matrix that allows to perpetuate the global health disparities rather than eradicating them, thereby reinforcing racialized narratives that position non-Western populations as sources of biological threat.

The pandemic has also illuminated the situational vulnerability of the racialized workforce, whose most vulnerable members were labelled as "essential workers" by the media, often romanticizing their precarious position. This new working class, distinguished by both heightened health risks and a simultaneous deprivation of adequate means of protection and subjected both to the dangers of viral exposure and the hovering threat of unemployment, reflects the shift from the classic Foucauldian sovereign's choice of "making live or letting die" to a coldly calculated differentiation between "lives worth risking" and "lives worth saving." This purely economic logic, forcing workers to choose between survival and employment, confirms that the boundary between political and physical life, as distinguished by conventional biopolitics, became increasingly blurred in response to the COVID-19 pandemic. Ultimately, it leads us back to the question of the usability and expendability of bodies, which, as Kandida Purnell's work has shown, is primarily determined on a racial basis in contemporary necropolitical frameworks, in which racialized populations are consumed, exploited and discarded without proper recognition of their suffering. As seen from the broader perspective, this supports Daniele Lorenzini's claim that today's biopolitics is still predominantly based on differential vulnerability, rooted in the need to maintain hierarchies and structural inequalities of populations to govern them. Focusing on individual responsibility in the face of a global pandemic shifts the blame onto victims of structural violence, obfuscating the role of biopolitics in shaping health and economic outcomes and thereby allowing us to avoid grappling with systemic racism by conveniently framing racial disparities as mere personal failings.

While the pandemic could have acted as an opportunity to address global racial injustices in healthcare, it seems unlikely for such an awakening to occur anytime soon. The same could be said about the capitalist logic underpinning the pandemic governance, as, despite calls for its modification, capitalism has demonstrated remarkable resilience, adapting its mechanisms to perpetuate racialized exploitation amidst global crises. Notwithstanding widespread protests against structural racial inequality and systemic injustice, COVID-19 has merely reinforced necropolitical regimes that extract and exploit racialized populations, resulting only in the exacerbation of existing inequalities. And despite a number of remedies proposed – decolonial, politico-economic, ecological, and solidary strategies – systemic racial inequalities remain deeply entrenched in the post-pandemic landscape, as the pandemic has exposed race-based faces of negative biopolitics and intensified the existing racial dynamics inherent to biopower, namely, the necropolitics of usable bodies and biopolitics based on the distribution of differential vulnerability.

Another contribution by J. D. Mininger, "Toward an Ethics of Dispossession: Philosophical Lessons from the Political Context of the COVID-19 Pandemic," offers an exploration of the intersection of mourning, critical reflexivity, and Foucauldian critique in the context of pandemic politics, emphasizing the importance of challenging power structures, advocating for ethical responses to the crisis. Imbued with critical reflexivity, the intricate process of mourning prompts an interrogation of power dynamics determining who is deemed worthy of it and who is not. Judith Butler's insights underscore the necessity of mourning as a means of identifying with suffering while critically evaluating the normative violence inherent in societal structures, whereas Michel Foucault's concept of critique, rooted in Kantian enlightenment ideals, advocates for ongoing self-transformation and resistance to dominant power structures. The author suggests that this critical ethos, aligned with virtue, challenges uncritical obedience and demands a reevaluation of governmentality and subjectivity in pandemic politics. By employing critical reflexivity and Foucauldian notion of critique in his reconsideration of mourning, J. D. Mininger formulates a call to action to subvert dominant narratives, resist normative violence, and foster a more equitable and just response to the pandemic's complexities.

In "The Death of Man: The Post-pandemic Condition?," Denis Petrina extends the critique of biopolitics by confronting its implicit anthropocentrism – an assumption that was profoundly unsettled during the pandemic. Foucault's prophetic image of man "erased like a face drawn in sand" serves as a conceptual departure point to interrogate what it means for the human to lose epistemological and ontological centrality in the wake of a planetary health crisis. While the literal demise of humanity may not have occurred, the epistemic destabilization of the human subject has been set in motion, thereby establishing a resonance between Foucault's work and posthumanist thought. The chapter contends that Foucault's writings, particularly his reflections on the body, already contain the seeds of posthuman biopolitics. The body emerges not as a stable and transparent entity but as ambivalent, porous, and epistemologically opaque. This latent dimension became starkly visible during the pandemic, as the *medical gaze* was internalized: that is to say, we came to perceive the obscurity within ourselves. Our bodies were exposed as fragile, leaky, and deeply dependent – not self-sufficient and autonomous, but inescapably entangled in heterogeneous assemblages with other bodies, masks, medicine, data flows, environments, and viral agents. This confrontation with our embodied incompleteness dislodges the illusion of humanist autonomy – an illusion ultimately linked to the emergence of the pandemic – and invites the development of post-anthropocentric politics attentive to the *more-than-human*.

This more-than-human biopolitics is unfolded through a close engagement with Foucault's key concepts – population, milieu, and governmentality, which, in the context of the pandemic, evolved into a form of *environmentality*. Rather than reinforcing the primacy of the human subject, these concepts illuminate a field of forces, processes, and interrelations. The cyber-dimension of pandemic management highlights this transformation: a hybrid regime of disciplinary techniques and algorithmic control reconfigures individuals into dividuals – datasets and epidemiological variables. What emerges here is the tectonic shift from classical anthropocentric biopolitics – the government of bodies – to what Lemke calls *the government of things* or computational biopolitics.

The chapter closes with a tentative sketch of the post-pandemic subject: no longer anchored in self-sufficiency but processually constituted through *technologies of the self*, attuned to ontological precarity, relationality, and care. Weaving together Foucault's late lectures with insights from posthumanist thinkers, the chapter calls to redefine health as *multispecies politics* – a horizon of collective, planetary entanglement. Here, the "death of man" is not a nihilistic conclusion, but the possibility for an ethics of radical healing, directed against the pathologies of human-centred epistemologies.

The anthropocentric premise of biopolitics is questioned in Audronė Žukauskaitė's article "Transindividual Biopolitics." The COVID-19 pandemic is interpreted as a biopolitical condition, which reveals that a human being is never a bounded individual but is always in relation to other human individuals and non-human beings, such as viruses. Moreover, a human being is dependent on technologies, such as new vaccines. It means that biopolitics should be understood not as an opposition between sovereign power and an individual but as an interaction between various individuals, technical objects, and natural forces. The article reintroduces the notion of the transindividual borrowed from the philosophies of Gilbert Simondon and Bernard Stiegler. The COVID-19 pandemic and the attempt to create a collective immunity (or "herd immunity") can be seen as a transindividual condition, where every individual is confronted with something pre-individual (namely, a virus) and, at the same time, with other individuals with whom it shares its immunity, thus creating a relationship of responsibility and solidarity. The transindividual can be reconsidered as a new mode of biopolitics: biopolitics is conceptualized not as a negative force but as an affirmative interaction between human and non-human forces and technological inventions. Such reconceptualization of biopolitics would change the focus from the opposition between a malicious power and subjugated individuals to the affirmative model of transindividual communities. It means that we might want to abandon the anthropocentric model of biopolitics and create a new one, that would embrace the biological and geo-biochemical conditions of the planet and the geological timescale of deep time.

The viability of conventional anthropocentric biopolitics is critically re-examined in Aistis Žekevičius' chapter "Post-pandemic Biopolitics: Reconciling the Geological, the Global, and the Planetary." The limitations of the Anthropocene studies, discussed by Kathryn Yusoff in their critique of the Anthropocene which emphasizes its material and colonial legacies, namely, its inability to address the racialized legacy of modernity, on the one hand, and understand race as a socio-geological construct that encompasses historically and culturally determined differences, on the other, underscore the urgency of adopting a biopolitical paradigm that would transcend anthropocentrism by acknowledging the interconnectedness of human and non-human lives and formations. From this perspective, the COVID-19 pandemic could be perceived as a catalyst for rethinking the mutual entanglement between biopolitical governance and the biosphere and reshaping governance structures to better account for planetary crises. The pandemic has equally exposed the inadequacies of existing political frameworks in responding to global crises of planetary extent, as the nation-states, deeply rooted in a territorial logic of governance, have struggled to respond to transnational crises that transcend conventional borders. To address these shortcomings, a shift toward planetary governance models that prioritize sustainability and ecological concerns is needed, and one of the possible solutions to ensure not only the sustainability but also the habitability of the planet could be reconciling the global and the planetary epistemes, as suggested by Dipesh Chakrabarty. Such a shift would entail moving beyond modernist paradigms that privilege economic growth and national sovereignty over the collective survival of both human and non-human species.

Last but not least, the pandemic has also demonstrated the importance of integrating the notions of care and reciprocity into the structures of biopower, which still tend to operate through a logic of control and extraction, to reconceptualize care as a planetary ethic that fosters coexistence rather than domination. As long as we seek to formulate a new biopolitical paradigm that focuses on care for both human and non-human beings, we should challenge anthropocentric governance models that prioritize short-term human economic interests over long-term strategies of planetary survival. Modernity has facilitated an epistemological framework that separates humans from nature, allowing us to treat the biosphere as an external resource to be managed rather than as an intrinsic part of political life. This separation of human and natural worlds has contributed to environmental degradation, systemic inequality, and governance failures in the face of global crises epitomized by COVID-19. In order to overcome these legacies, a fundamental restructuring of biopolitical thought is needed, one that would integrate ecological and planetary perspectives into governance by embracing indigenous knowledge systems, relational ontologies, and holistic approaches to sustainability. While the prospects for equitable and realistic planetary biopolitics in a post-pandemic world remain highly unlikely, the proposed notion of geoplanetary biopolitics offers plenty of potential in overcoming the limitations of conventional biopolitics by acknowledging the historical links between colonialism, capitalism and racialization and considering the ecological and technological aspects of contemporary biogovernance from a planetary viewpoint. "Post-pandemic Biopolitics" is an attempt to resolve this necropolitical impasse by emphasizing the pressing need to move beyond conventional anthropocentric biopolitics and offering the outlines of a new multi-scale paradigm that would acknowledge the interconnectedness of human and non-human life and propose a process-oriented reconceptualization of race.

Finally, Audronė Žukauskaitė's article "Immunity and Symbiopolitics examines the relationship between human and non-human worlds. The recent COVID-19 pandemic exposed the urgent need to create collective immunity, or "herd immunity," and, thus, rethink the dialectics between immunity and community. Although immunity is usually seen as the perfect metaphor for biopolitical government, which fights everything it sees as "non-self," its mode of operation is twofold. As seen from the perspective of contemporary biology, immunity comprises not only a defensive reaction toward an external, contagious element but also a positive reaction or the so-called "tolerance." Alfred I. Tauber suggested that immunity should be seen as an ecological system that not merely reacts to the external element but opens the negotiations between the "self" and "non-self" within the system. Ecological immunity, therefore, helps to rethink the notion of biopolitics; instead of seeing biopolitics as the opposition between a sovereign power and an oppressed individual, we can interpret it as a network of sympoietic interactions between human and non-human individuals. This allows us to argue that every biopolitics is always already symbiopolitics, affecting the conditions of liveability of both human and non-human symbionts. As Latour pointed out, this kind of symbiosis can be seen not only in the recent pandemic situation when humans have to fight against viruses but also in the recent ecological crisis when humanity itself acts as a virulent pathogen that keeps changing the conditions of liveability. The model of symbiopolitics reveals that every individual always already acts as a community, composed of both an internal ecosystem and an external ecosystem, co-functioning with human and non-human others. Such an affirmative model of symbiopolitics reframes the opposition between immunity and community: to acquire immunity, I do not have to protect the "self" from "non-self" or "other"; on the contrary, the "other" is what makes "my" immunity possible. Thus, the notion of symbiopolitics allows us to conceptualize differences and heterogeneities in a positive way.

These "discontents with biopolitics" encourage us to think about different approaches which could operate on local, global, and planetary scales. The old conventional biopolitics persists because deep-seated social, racial, or geopolitical inequalities do not simply disappear; moreover, most of them seem to be structurally inseparable from the functioning of biopolitics as such. However, this conventional biopolitics should be supplemented with what we call planetary biopolitics, which encompasses both ecological and technological dimensions of contemporary governmentality. It does not mean that conventional biopolitics should be abandoned; rather, it means that biopolitics should reconsider the legacies of colonialism and imperialism and acknowledge its effects on recent regimes of racialization and extractivism in the Anthropocene. Biopolitics is not only the extraction of labor-force but also the extraction of biological and geological life on a planetary scale. This, in turn, encourages us to formulate the notion of planetary biopolitics, which would take into account all forms of human life (racialized, Indigenous, neglected life), all forms of biological life (biological diversity), and geological life of different complexity (water, atmosphere, the earth). Planetary biopolitics should acknowledge that the governance of life no longer aligns with national borders and operates on different – local, global, and planetary – scales.

Index

www.ingramcontent.com/pod-product-compliance
Lightning Source LLC
Chambersburg PA
CBHW051401240926
51852CB00002B/86
9789004748170